MISSION MEDICAL FINALS

Neurology + Psychiatry
EMQs & OSCEs

Authors
Dr Neil Wellappili MBBS BSc
Dr Kumaran Saha MBBS
Mr Ranbir Sandhu MBBS MA (Cantab) MRCS

Editor
Dr Michael De Souza MBBS BSc

Editorial advisors
Neurology: Dr Paul J Hughes RD, QHP, MD, FRCP
Psychiatry: Dr Peter Raven MBBS PhD MRCP MRCPsych

With special thanks to Dr Samantha Wellappili MBBS

Published by ISC Medical (www.iscmedical.co.uk)

First Edition: July 2009
ISBN13: 978-1-905812-08-0
A catalogue record for this book is available from the British Library.

Printed in the United Kingdom by:
Aidan's Ltd. Reg. Office, 35 Ballards Lane, London N3 1XW

The authors have, as far as possible, taken care to ensure that the information given in this text is accurate and up to date at time of publication. The information within this text is intended as a study aid for the purpose of the medical school examinations. It is not intended, nor should it be used as a medical reference for the direct management of patients or their conditions. Readers are strongly advised to confirm that the information with regards to specific patient management complies with current legislation, guidelines and local protocols.

About the Authors

Between us, we studied at University College, Bart's and Cambridge medical schools. We are currently working in Foundation jobs. We remember as students how challenging neuroscience can be and our focus in writing this book has been to provide candidates with clear and comprehensive explanations.

Revising for our finals, we benefited from working together, particularly OSCE scenarios. One of the best ways to learn, which we discovered to our cost, is to fall on your face. We arrived at the study techniques outlined in the following pages through our mishaps; using them to learn common neuroscience conditions will help you get through your medical school exams more smoothly. We all comfortably passed our clinical neuroscience exams, one with a merit (he doesn't like to boast though).

About the Editorial Advisors

Dr Paul Hughes studied medicine at the Welsh National School of Medicine. He was appointed Consultant Neurologist at Hurstwood Park Neurological Hospital In 1994. He is a Surgeon Captain in the Royal Naval Reserve and is the Specialist Adviser in Neurology to the Royal Navy.

Dr Peter Raven studied medicine at University College London. He is the Faculty Tutor (Biomedical Sciences) and Deputy Director of Medical Education at the Royal Free and University College Medical School as well as an honorary consultant psychiatrist for Camden and Islington Mental Health Trust.

Contents

EMQs

OSCEs

REFERENCES

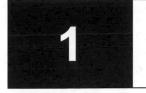

Introduction to EMQs

FORMAT

Extended matching questions (EMQs) are used increasingly in medical exams, including finals. Each question typically consists of 5 scenarios, for which the student should select the best answer from 10 options.

Most EMQ-based exams last up to 3 hours and allow students up to 1 minute to answer each scenario. In this book we have provided 100 neurology scenarios and 100 psychiatry scenarios. You should aim to complete each set of 100 scenarios in 1 hour and 40 minutes.

EXAM TIPS

At the start at the exam, try to scan through the whole paper in a few minutes. When you reach questions you can't answer, mark them in pencil and return to them later. It will stop you procrastinating, and falling behind, with the risk of missing out on easier questions near the end. Aim to finish with at least ten minutes to spare in which to check your answers. Avoid staying up late the night before, as you won't be sharp enough to spot your mistakes.

When you read a scenario for the first time, try to visualize the answer before reading the options, as these can be misleading. Many scenarios hinge on the recognition of key phrases such as "Kernig's sign" (pathognomic of meningitis). When you are not able to visualise the answer, you might instead be able to exclude several options at first glance.

Some options may be used more than once in a single EMQ; check if this is mentioned in each question or at the start of the paper. Even when this is allowed, an option is repeated less often than would be expected on chance alone. Therefore think carefully before using one of the options twice. In this book we explain all the options presented and reveal the mechanics behind EMQs.

When reading EMQ scenarios - as in medical practice - consider the odds ratio (OR). This is the probability that a new symptom is caused by a condition the patient is known to have (P1), divided by the chance that they have another disease (P2) and that this is causing the symptom (P3) i.e. OR = P1/ (P2 x P3). This illustrates why unusual complications of rare conditions that the patient has already been diagnosed with are often more likely than new presentations of separate common conditions. Thus, in a person known to have untreated HIV, cognitive impairment and upper motor neurone signs are more likely to be caused by a CNS infection such as a toxoplasma abscess than by them having had a cerebrovascular accident presenting in the same fashion.

REVISION TECHNIQUES

EMQs test knowledge of different aspects of medicine, be it aetiology, management, complications or other factors. You might find it useful to learn common conditions according to a standard framework, as outlined in this mnemonic:-

Doctors	→	**Definition**
R	→	**Risk factors**
Always	→	**Aetiology**
Emphasising	→	**Epidemiology**
History and	→	**History**
Examination	→	**Examination**
In	→	**Investigations**
Management of	→	**Management**
Clinical	→	**Complications**
Problems	→	**Prognosis**
Daily	→	**Differential diagnosis**

 Look out for further mnemonics throughout this book, devised to aid your revision, marked by this symbol.

2 Neurology EMQs

| 1 | Headache | NEUROLOGY |

Options

A   Angle-closure glaucoma
B   Cerebrovascular accident
C   Cluster headache
D   Giant cell arteritis
E   Idiopathic intracranial hypertension
F   Meningitis
G   Sagittal sinus thrombosis
H   Space-occupying lesion
I   Subarachnoid haemorrhage
J   Trigeminal neuralgia

Select the most appropriate diagnosis from the list above (each may be used once or more)

1.   A 72-year-old woman with weight loss, pain on chewing, left-sided headache, shoulder pain and sudden visual loss.

2.   A 44-year-old man with bouts of right-sided headache, painful red eye and lacrimation lasting hours. His pupils are normal.

3.   A 19-year-old obese woman with generalised headache and papilloedema that is worse in the morning and is alleviated by cerebrospinal fluid drainage.

4.   A 25-year-old man with post-coital "thunderclap" headache, photophobia, neck stiffness and vomiting.

5.   A 22-year-old woman with cystic acne and onset of left sided hemiplegia and right-sided headache after coughing.

| 2 | Headache | NEUROLOGY |

Options
A   Cerebrovascular accident
B   Dural sinus thrombosis
C   Dural tear
D   Meningitis
E   Migraine
F   Space-occupying lesion
G   Subarachnoid haemorrhage
H   Subdural haemorrhage
I   Trigeminal neuralgia
J   None of the above

Select the most appropriate diagnosis from the list above (each may be used once or more).

6.   A 3-month-old febrile infant with poor handling, blanching macular rash, fever and positive Kernig's sign.

7.   A 41-year-old man with a broken cheekbone following an assault, whose headache is worse when upright.

8.   A 22-year-old woman with headache worse in the morning, vomiting and Cushing reflex.

9.   An 18-year-old febrile man with headache, rigors, leg pain and blanching macular rash.

10. A 72-year-old woman with a headache, confusion and drowsiness that worsen in the evening, with gradual onset over the last few winter months.

| 3 | Lumbar puncture | NEUROLOGY |

Options
A   Acute disseminated encephalomyelitis
B   Bacterial meningitis
C   Cerebral toxoplasmosis
D   Carcinomatous meningitis
E   Fungal meningitis
F   Multiple sclerosis
G   Neurosyphilis
H   Progressive multifocal leucoencephalopathy
I   Tuberculous meningitis
J   Viral meningitis

Select the most appropriate diagnosis from the list above (each may be used once or more).

11. A 22-year-old man with headache, fever and drowsiness. CSF lymphocytes are 193/mm³, glucose 4mM, protein 0.8g/litre. Blood glucose is 7.8mM.

12. A 27-year-old woman with headache, weight loss, fever and drowsiness. CSF lymphocytes are 92/mm³, protein 0.75g/litre, glucose concentration 3.1mM and positivity for Indian ink stain. Blood glucose is 6.9mM.

13. A 34-year-old woman with relapsing-remitting eye pain, l'Hermitte's sign and exaggerated tendon reflexes. CSF lymphocytes are 24/mm³, glucose 4mM, protein 0.9g/litre, oligoclonal IgG bands on electrophoresis. Blood glucose is 6mM.

14. A 31-year-old man with confusion, clonus and exaggerated reflexes. CSF lymphocytes are 23/mm³, glucose 4.5mM, protein 0.7g/litre, PCR positive for JC virus. Blood glucose is 7.3mM.

15. A 43-year-old man with headache, weight loss, fever and drowsiness. CSF lymphocytes are 504/mm³, glucose 2.8mM, protein 3.1g/litre. Blood glucose is 6.6mM. Ziehl-Neelsen stain of CSF is positive.

4	Red eye	NEUROLOGY

Options
A	Anterior uveitis
B	Angle closure glaucoma
C	Bacterial conjunctivitis
D	Cavernous sinus thrombosis
E	Conjunctival haemorrhage
F	Graves' disease
G	Keratitis
H	Sjogren's syndrome
I	Subconjunctival haemorrhage
J	Trachoma

Select the most appropriate diagnosis from the list above (each may be used once or more).

16. A 52-year-old long-sighted man with a red and painful right eye who sees haloes around street lights in the rain. The pain is worse when he is in the cinema. His pupil is dilated and lacks a light response.

17. A 35-year-old woman with fever, headache, an oedematous right eyelid, diplopia, red eye, proptosis and impaired corneal reflex.

18. A 31-year-old man with bilateral red eye and crusting. Acuity, pupillary reflexes and intraocular pressure are normal.

19. A 36-year-old woman with sudden pain and positive Talbot's test in one eye. The pupil is small, with lacrimation, pain on looking at light and impaired vision. On x-ray, she has "bamboo spine".

20. An 8-year-old boy with bilateral follicular inflammation.

| 5 | Motor symptoms | NEUROLOGY |

Options

A   Becker's muscular dystrophy
B   Cauda equina syndrome
C   Common peroneal nerve palsy
D   Dermatomyositis
E   Diabetic neuropathy
F   Duchenne's muscular dystrophy
G   Guillain-Barré syndrome
H   Myasthenia gravis
I   Spinal cord compression
J   Tibial nerve palsy

Select the most appropriate diagnosis from the list above (each may be used once or more).

21. A 65-year-old woman with violaceous rash on her eyelids and shoulder girdle weakness.

22. A 31-year-old woman with backache, sciatica, leg weakness and absent plantar reflex.

23. A 33-year-old woman recovering from pneumonia, with respiratory compromise and leg weakness.

24. A 38-year-old woman with right-sided footdrop following a fibula fracture.

25. A 6-year-old boy with clumsy walking, Gower's sign and large calves.

6	Motor symptoms	NEUROLOGY

Options

A   Anterior cerebral artery cerebrovascular accident
B   Bulbar palsy
C   Guillain-Barré syndrome
D   Middle cerebral artery cerebrovascular accident
E   Motor neurone disease
F   Multiple sclerosis
G   Spinal cord compression
H   Subacute combined degeneration of the spinal cord
I   Syringobulbia
J   None of the above

Select the most appropriate diagnosis from the list above (each may be used once or more).

26.   A 28-year-old woman with dysphagia, absent gag reflex, amyotrophy of the arms, exaggerated right ankle and knee reflexes, with loss of pain and temperature sensation bilaterally at her scalp, chin, ears, neck, shoulders and arms.

27.   A 24-year-old man with dysphagia, absent gag reflex, tongue fasciculations, ankle clonus, muscle wasting, and exaggerated ankle, bicep and knee reflexes.

28.   A 32-year-old woman with rigidity, exaggerated ankle, biceps and knee jerks, with Chvostek's sign following neck surgery.

29.   A 73-year-old man with sudden onset of left leg and arm weakness, exaggerated left ankle, knee and biceps reflexes, though his arm is affected less severely.

30.   A 50-year-old confused woman with Hashimoto's thyroiditis, exaggerated knee reflexes, absent ankle reflexes and bilateral upwards plantar reflex.

| 7 | Neurological emergencies | NEUROLOGY |

Options

A   Bacterial meningitis
B   Cerebral malaria
C   Cerebrovascular accident
D   Extradural haemorrhage
E   Fibromuscular dysplasia
F   Giant cell arteritis
G   Status epilepticus
H   Subdural haemorrhage
I   Toxoplasmosis
J   Transient ischemic attack

Select the most appropriate diagnosis from the list above (each may be used once or more).

31. A 63-year-old confused man with fever, headache worse on waking, papilloedema, diarrhoea, seizures, weight loss and paresis in his right arm.

32. A 40-year-old mercenary with tertian fever, headache, cyanosis, tachypnoea and upward plantar response.

33. An 80-year-old woman with recent onset weakness on the left side of her face, her left arm and leg, with exaggerated reflexes and up-ward plantar response.

34. A 47-year-old alcoholic man with impaired consciousness, Cushing's reflex and vomiting.

35. A 31-year-old man who was knocked unconscious by a cricket ball. He recovered then collapsed after the match.

8	CNS infection	NEUROLOGY

Options
A   Brown-Séquard syndrome
B   Cerebral malaria
C   Meningococcal septicaemia
D   Progressive multifocal leucoencephalopathy
E   Tabes dorsalis
F   Taboparesis
G   Toxoplasmosis abscess
H   Tuberculoma
I   Viral encephalitis
J   Viral meningitis

Select the most appropriate diagnosis from the list above (each may be used once or more).

36.   An 18-year-old woman with fever, vomiting, severe thigh pain, cold hands and cold feet.

37.   A 25-year-old man with exaggerated left knee and ankle reflexes, with loss of proprioception and vibroception on his left leg. His right leg is unaffected apart from loss of pain and temperature sensation.

38.   A 7-year-old Burmese girl with gradual regression of developmental markers, upward plantar response and myoclonic seizures.

39.   A 62-year-old man with ataxia, stamping unsteady gait, bilateral loss of knee and ankle reflexes and "lightning pains" in his legs.

40.   A 2-year-old boy who cannot walk or speak, with extensor plantar response, exaggerated reflexes and Argyll Robertson pupils.

| 9 | **Treatment of Parkinsonian symptoms** | **NEUROLOGY** |

Options

A   Apomorphine and domperidone
B   Benserazide
C   Benzhexol
D   Bromocriptine
E   Entacapone
F   Levodopa
G   Pergolide
H   Ropinerole
I   Selegiline
J   None of the above

Select the most appropriate drug from the list above (each may be used once or more).

41.   Dopa-decarboxylase inhibitor given to minimise peripheral effects of dopamine.

42.   Enzyme inhibitor used to delay the need for treatment with levodopa.

43.   Given as subcutaneous infusion for management of severe on-off effects in advanced Parkinson's disease.

44.   Given for treatment of severe tremor, may cause confusion.

45.   Given alongside levodopa and entacapone.

10	Peripheral neuropathy	NEUROLOGY

Options

A   Cervical rib syndrome
B   Charcot-Marie-Tooth syndrome
C   Chlorambucil-induced neuropathy
D   Meralgia paraesthetica
E   Leprosy
F   Mononeuritis multiplex
G   Radial nerve palsy
H   Tuberculosis
I   Ulnar nerve palsy
J   Vincristine-induced neuropathy

Select the most appropriate diagnosis from the list above (each may be used once or more).

46. A 22-year-old man with acute lymphoblastic leukaemia experiences constipation with tingling in his feet and hands.

47. A 25-year-old pregnant woman with numbness of her anterior thigh.

48. A 19-year-old woman with left forearm pain, numbness in the axilla and medial upper arm with wasting of the left hand.

49. A 31-year-old man with weakness of the extensor digitorum, wrist-drop, impaired triceps jerk and weakness of thumb extension.

50. A 26-year-old man with footdrop, thenar wasting, wristdrop and numb, pale skin lesions.

| 11 | Treatment of CNS infection | NEUROLOGY |

Options
A Intramuscular benzylpenicillin
B Intramuscular benzylpenicillin and intravenous cefotaxime
C Intravenous aciclovir
D Intravenous co-trimoxazole
E Intravenous flucytosine and amphotericin
F Oral cefotaxime
G Oral ciprofloxacin
H Oral erythromycin
I Oral rifampicin
J Oral sulphadiazine, pyrimethamine, folinic acid

Select the most appropriate treatment from the list above (each may be used once or more).

51. A 15-year-old girl with rapidly worsening illness causing fever, cold peripheries, non-blanching rash, neck stiffness and photophobia.

52. A 35-year-old HIV-positive woman has fever, reduced consciousness and an Indian ink staining organism on lumbar puncture. What treatment, in addition to antiretrovirals, is required?

53. A 42-year-old man with recent onset of seizures. Lumbar puncture finds a lymphocytosis, while EEG shows periodic complexes. What treatment, in addition to anti-epileptic medication, is needed?

54. A 22-year-old woman whose boyfriend has bacterial meningitis. She takes the oral contraceptive pill.

55. A 47-year-old HIV-positive man with ring-shaped contrast-enhancing lesions on CT scan. What treatment, in addition to antiretrovirals, is required?

12	Epilepsy treatment	NEUROLOGY

Options

A   Intravenous carbamazepine
B   Intravenous phenytoin
C   Intravenous thiopentone and assisted ventilation
D   Oral carbamazepine
E   Oral clobazam
F   Oral clonazepam
G   Oral gabapentin
H   Oral lamotrigine
I   Oral phenytoin
J   Oral sodium valproate

Select the most appropriate treatment from the list above (each may be used once or more).

56. A 29-year-old woman with partial seizures in which she hears odd sounds. She is taking the oral contraceptive pill for polycystic ovarian syndrome.

57. A 23-year-old woman with seizures during which she becomes unresponsive and pale for a few seconds. EEG shows bilateral 3Hz spike and slow wave complexes. She is trying to become pregnant.

58. A 13-year-old girl with brief jerks of the arms and legs, particularly in the morning, sometimes followed by whole-body seizures with loss of consciousness. She is jaundiced due to hepatitis A.

59. A 15-year-old boy with seizures in which he falls to the floor, tense and unconscious before shaking violently for up to 2 minutes, during which he is incontinent. He has a history of bone marrow depression.

60. A 9-year-old boy with onset of violent seizures with incontinence, unconsciousness and no intervening recovery that has so far lasted 10 minutes. What medication is required in addition to basic life support and oxygen?

| 13 | Cranial nerve palsy | NEUROLOGY |

Options

A   II nerve
B   left XI nerve
C   left XII nerve
D   right XII nerve
E   right XI nerve
F   VII lower motor neurone lesion
G   VII upper motor neurone lesion
H   V/VII/VIII/IX nerve
I   V/VII/VIII nerve
J   V/VI/VII nerve

Select the most appropriate diagnosis from the list above (each may be used once or more).

61. A 54-year-old woman presents to her GP, unable to move her head to the left and shrug her right shoulder.

62. A 68-year-old man's tongue deviates to the left when he sticks it out.

63. A 61-year-old woman with left-sided facial weakness sparing the occipitofrontalis muscle.

64. A 31-year-old woman with paradoxical left-sided pupillary dilatation on the swinging light test.

65. A 52-year-old man presents with gradual deafness and dizziness with weakness and numbness on the same side of the face.

14	Predisposing factors	NEUROLOGY

Options

A Cocaine use
B Country of origin
C Hypertension
D Polycystic kidney disease
E Positive family history
F Poverty
G Prematurity
H Septal defect
I Sickle cell disease
J Splenectomy

Select the most appropriate predisposing factor from the list above (each may be used once or more).

66. Following a 14-hour plane journey, a 37-year-old man suddenly develops weakness and reduced tone in his right arm and leg.

67. A 31-year-old woman, who previously survived a serious car crash, develops cold peripheries, rigors and thigh pain.

68. A 35-year-old woman develops muscle weakness and paraesthesia. She had a previous episode of painful visual disturbance.

69. A 45-year-old man with longstanding left wrist contracture.

70. A 42-year-old man with recent onset of jerky uncontrollable semi-disguised purposeless movements and personality change.

| 15 | Aetiology of dyskinesias | NEUROLOGY |

Options

A   Athetoid cerebral palsy
B   Essential tremor
C   Hemiballismus
D   Huntington's chorea
E   Parkinson's disease
F   Primary torsion dystonia
G   Sydenham's chorea
H   Tourette's syndrome
I   Wilson's disease
J   None of the above

Select the most appropriate condition to fit the aetiology, from the list above (each may be used once or more).

71.   Acetylcholine and gamma-aminobutyric acid secretion from the corpus striatum is impaired, causing unintentional movements.

72.   Defects at the cerebellum causing an inherited movement disorder.

73.   Infarct at the left subthalamic nucleus causing unintentional movements.

74.   Eosinophilic inclusion bodies present at the substantia nigra pars compacta causing rigidity and akinesia.

75.   Serum caeruloplasmin protein is low, brown-yellow rings are seen on the cornea; rigidity and akinesia are present.

16	Causes of seizures	NEUROLOGY

Options

A Disseminated intravascular coagulation
B Drug withdrawal
C Fever
D Hypokalemia
E Hyponatremia
F Hypoxia
G Idiopathic epilepsy
H Neurocysticercosis
I   Pseudoseizure
J   Type 1 neurofibromatosis

Select the most appropriate answer from the list above (each may be used once or more).

76. A 22-year-old woman with 8 brown "café-au-lait" spots, Lisch nodules on slit lamp fundoscopy and shaking fits.

77. A 32-year-old depressed man collapses and shakes on the floor, with incontinence and tongue-biting.

78. A 9-year-old Spanish boy with headache, vomiting, papilloedema and seizures.

79. A 29-year-old man hallucinates about spiders on the floor before undergoing violent convulsions.

80. An 18-year-old febrile woman with widespread ecchymoses, hypotension and tachycardia loses consciousness and shakes.

| 17 | CNS tumours | NEUROLOGY |

Options

A Acoustic neuroma
B Astrocytoma
C Ependymoma
D Glioblastoma multiforme
E Lymphoma
F Medulloblastoma
G Meningioma
H Oligodendroglioma
I Pituitary adenoma
J Retinoblastoma

Select the most appropriate diagnosis from the list above (each may be used once or more).

81. A 24-year-old man with bilateral sensorineural hearing loss and vertigo.

82. A 12-year-old girl with vertigo, ataxia, nausea and a mass in her fourth ventricle.

83. A 53-year-old man with Kernohan grade IV malignant tumour of the frontal lobe.

84. A 39-year-old man with tingling pain in both of his hands, prognathism, diabetes and visual field defects.

85. A 1-year-old boy with a white instead of red pupil reflex.

| 18 | Cognitive impairment | NEUROLOGY |

Options

A   Alzheimer's dementia
B   Colloid cyst
C   Creutzfeldt-Jakob disease
D   Folate deficiency
E   Frontotemporal dementia
F   HIV encephalopathy
G   Huntington's chorea
H   Multi-infarct dementia
I   Lewy body dementia
J   Parkinson's disease

Select the most appropriate diagnosis from the list above (each may be used once or more).

86. A 41-year-old man with declining cognition, headache, urinary incontinence, paraesthesia in both legs and unsteady gait.

87. A 74-year-old man with labile mood, deteriorating memory, fluent nonsensical speech, anomia and positive grasp reflex.

88. An 80-year-old man with micrographia, an inexpressive face, shuffling gait, resting tremor and progressive memory impairment.

89. A 78-year-old man with a long history of smoking, progressive cognitive deterioration and spasticity in his right arm.

90. A 77-year-old man with spatial disorientation and gradually worsening memory. Apart from during transient lucid intervals, he cannot recognise his carers and believes that his care home is his house.

19	Visual loss	NEUROLOGY

Options

- A   Amblyopia
- B   Central retinal vein thrombosis
- C   Hypertensive retinopathy
- D   Macular degeneration
- E   Parietal lobe CVA
- F   Retinal detachment
- G   Retinitis pigmentosa
- H   Retrobulbar neuritis
- I   Temporal lobe CVA
- J   Vitamin A deficiency

Select the most appropriate diagnosis from the list above (each may be used once or more).

91. A 69-year-old man has progressively worsening vision over the last 6 months. On fundoscopy, his GP notices grey-yellow spots at the back of the eye.

92. A 44-year-old man with blurred vision, retinal flame haemorrhages, disc swelling without venous pulsation and bilaterally enlarged blind spots.

93. A 40-year-old man who describes sporadically seeing bright shapes in the centre of his visual field, burning white "like the Sun".

94. A 37-year-old woman with unilateral impaired central vision and eye pain on movement. Fundoscopy is normal.

95. A 64-year-old woman with bilateral loss of vision in the right lower quadrant.

| 20 | Treatment of pain syndromes | NEUROLOGY |

Options
A   Carbamazepine
B   Codeine
C   Fentanyl
D   Gabapentin
E   Ketamine
F   Morphine
G   Paracetamol and sumatriptan
H   Prednisolone and alendronic acid
I   Sumatriptan
J   Tolfenamic acid

Select the most appropriate treatment from the list above (each may be used once or more).

96. A 58-year-old diabetic man with burning pain in his feet.

97. A 69-year-old woman with left-sided facial pain and amaurosis fugax.

98. A 71-year-old man with breakthrough lower back pain and disseminated prostate cancer.

99. A 33-year-old woman with intense bursts of left-sided facial pain lasting seconds.

100. An 8-year-old girl about to enter the operating theatre prior to an appendicectomy.

3 Neurology EMQs Answers & Explanations

Quick Answers

1	D	2	C	3	E	4	I	5	G
6	D	7	C	8	F	9	D	10	J
11	J	12	E	13	F	14	H	15	I
16	B	17	D	18	C	19	A	20	J
21	D	22	B	23	G	24	C	25	F
26	I	27	E	28	J	29	A	30	H
31	I	32	B	33	C	34	H	35	D
36	C	37	A	38	I	39	E	40	F
41	B	42	I	43	A	44	C	45	B
46	J	47	D	48	A	49	G	50	E
51	B	52	E	53	C	54	G	55	J
56	H	57	H	58	H	59	J	60	B
61	E	62	C	63	G	64	A	65	I
66	H	67	J	68	B	69	G	70	E
71	D	72	B	73	C	74	E	75	I
76	J	77	E	78	H	79	B	80	A
81	A	82	C	83	D	84	I	85	J
86	B	87	E	88	I	89	H	90	A
91	D	92	C	93	F	94	H	95	E
96	D	97	H	98	C	99	A	100	E

Explanations

1 – D

Jaw claudication (painful chewing due to muscle ischaemia), **amaurosis fugax** (sudden visual loss) and the patient's **advanced age** strongly suggest **giant cell arteritis** (AKA temporal arteritis). Other causes of persistent severe headache in an older person include tension headache, Paget's disease of the skull and cervical spondylosis.

2 – C

The **duration** is key. **Cluster headaches** occur in bursts lasting 15-150 **minutes**, while trigeminal neuralgia bursts last seconds. As the pupil is normal, angle-closure glaucoma can be excluded.

3 – E

Only **idiopathic intracranial hypertension** would respond to **therapeutic CSF drainage**. However, this is hazardous in initial diagnosis, because other causes of intracranial hypertension can cause death by brainstem coning on lumbar puncture (CT scans would be required to exclude this risk). Idiopathic intracranial hypertension occurs with a lack of localising signs and all investigations except CSF pressure being normal. Prevalence is increased in young, obese women and there is an association with oral contraceptive and tetracycline usage. Other therapeutic options include thiazide diuretics, acetazolamide, frusemide, prednisolone and weight loss. If these fail, surgical treatments include ventriculoperitoneal shunts, lumboperitoneal shunts and optic nerve fenestration.

4 – I

"**Thunderclap**" is the key word, emphasizing a sudden devastating pain, which (particularly without rash or fever) suggests **subarachnoid haemorrhage** over meningitis.

5 – G

The mention of **severe acne** is key, as skin infections can lead to **dural sinus thrombosis** via emissary veins through the skull, connecting scalp veins and the superior sagittal sinus. Most headaches are worsened by **coughing,** but when this induces a headache, secondary causes are suggested. Although this is a form of CVA, **G** is more specific. Sinus thrombosis can be differentiated from arterial stroke by neuro-imaging and D-dimer estimation. Predisposing factors include prothrombotic blood disorders, pregnancy, septicaemia, contraceptive pill use, diabetes and dehydration. CVA is suggested by headache on the contralateral side to hemiparaesthesia or hemiparesis.

Further Information (Q. 1 – 5)

Red flags are clinical features indicating serious disease. With headache, these include **"first and worst headache"** (suspect subarachnoid haemorrhage), **headache with fever and a rash** (suspect meningitis), **excruciating eye pain and headache** (suspect acute angle closure glaucoma), **jaw claudication and visual loss** (suspect giant cell arteritis). Signs of raised intracranial pressure are red flags for space occupying lesions-headache induced by coughing, hypertension and bradycardia (Cushing's reflex), headache worse when lying down (e.g.in the morning) and straining, papilloedema, fits, false localising signs (e.g. VI nerve palsy), focal signs (e.g. leg weakness), irregular (Cheyne-Stokes) respiration, reduced consciousness, vomiting.

---

6 – D

There should be a low threshold for diagnosing **meningitis** or meningococcal septicaemia, particularly with infants. The absence of the classic non-blanching (i.e. haemorrhagic) petechial rash doesn't exclude it-blanching rash can result from meningococcal septicaemia in the first 24 hours of onset, the non-blanching rash tending to develop subsequently. Even later, as blood vessels are further damaged, large ecchymotic non-blanching rashes (bruising) may form, signalling the risk of gangrene. A positive **Kernig's sign** occurs when straightening the patient's knee while their hip is extended causes painful spasms. Other features of meningism include **Brudzinski's sign**, whereby passively flexing the neck of a supine patient causes them to involuntarily lift their legs. Meningitis may also cause a high-pitched moaning cry, neck retraction, tense fontanelles (due to raised intracranial pressure), rigors, poor responsiveness, abnormal tone, cyanosis, and poor feeding in infants. In older people, it may cause photophobia, a stiff neck and acute confusional state.

7 – C

The key point is that the pain is **worse when upright**- due to more CSF leaking. **Dural tears** over the cribriform plate of the ethmoid bone can cause CSF rhinorrhoea, which can be diagnosed with urine dipsticks (CSF but not mucus tests positive for glucose). CSF leaks may cause brainstem herniation and are further investigated by MRI. Treatments include bedrest, hydration and caffeine IV. Morphine may have to be avoided with head injuries because it causes pinpoint pupils, preventing the testing of brainstem function by pupil reflexes.

8 – F

Cushing reflex and headache **worse in the morning** are key signs because they both suggest **raised intracranial pressure**. Cushing reflex is hypertension and bradycardia, cardiovascular adaptations to maintain cerebral bloodflow despite raised intracranial pressure. The headache is worse on waking because lying down increases intracranial pressure.

9 – D

All these features suggest **meningitis**, even in the absence of the classic non-blanching rash.

10 – J

The key is the **season**; this is **carbon monoxide toxicity**, caused by poorly ventilated heaters. Space-occupying lesions cause headache worst on waking as opposed to at the end of the day. It is important to ask about gas heating at home, specifically the presence of soot and orange flames. Carbon monoxide displaces oxygen from haemoglobin molecules and compromises the oxygenation of brain cells. Haemoglobin saturation by pulse oximetry is normal, though oxygen potential pressure is low on ABG, Advanced cases may cause cherry-red mucous membranes.

Further Information (Q. 6 – 10)

Incidence of **bacterial meningitis** is 5-10 per 100 000 per year in the UK, with risk factors including immunocompromise, splenectomy, alcoholism, sickle cell disease, diabetes mellitus, CSF shunts, poverty, overcrowding and basal skull fracture. Spina bifida occulta malformation and basal skull fractures can cause recurrent meningitis.

The two main age groups affected in the UK are children under 5 and 15-19-year-olds, with peak presentation in winter. Infants in the UK are vaccinated against Meningococcus C and H. Influenza B, travellers to high-incidence areas in the Tropics require Meningococcus C and A vaccinations, whilst Hajj or Umrah pilgrims travelling to Saudi Arabia require the ACWY (for types A,C,Y and W135) meningococcal vaccine.

The Meningitis Research Foundation recommends that all children with fever and non-blanching rash should be given IV antibiotics. Meningococcus causes combined meningitis and septicaemia in more than 50% of cases, septicaemia alone in more than 30%, while fewer than 15% result in meningitis alone (Campbell and Cranfield 1996). Non-blanching rash isn't encountered with M. Tuberculosis and H. Influenzae meningitis, and only develops (late) in ~50% of meningococcal meningitis cases. Yung and McDonald (2003) advise that 2 or more of the following early cues suggest meningococcal septicaemia:

- Non-blanching rash;
- Blanching macular or maculopapular rash (more easily seen on the palms and soles of darker skin);
- Contact with another infected person;
- Vomiting in a previously healthy person without diarrhoea;
- Severe muscle pain in neck, back or limbs- particularly anterior thigh;
- Clinical features in a child severe enough to cause serious concern from carers;
- Rapidly worsening symptoms.

Septicaemia and meningitis can each be fatal- meningitis by CNS failure, septicaemia by cardiovascular failure. Bacterial meningitis has a mortality rate of 70-100% if untreated (meningococcal meningitis has a ~15% mortality in the UK overall). Viral meningitis tends to be self-limiting in immunocompetent individuals but can present in a similar fashion to viral encephalitis, which has a ~70% mortality rate without treatment (~20% with treatment).

---

11 – J
Viral meningitis is suggested by lymphocytosis, raised protein and normal glucose, combined with no detectable organism on microscopy or culture of the CSF. Viral meningitis tends to be self-limiting, though it can present with the same symptoms as viral encephalitis, which may be fatal and requires antiviral treatment.

12 – E
Positive **Indian ink stain** is diagnostic of the **Cryptococcus** fungus. Cryptococcal meningitis is an AIDS-defining illness (i.e. diagnosis marks the onset of AIDS in an HIV-positive person), with onset when CD4 lymphocyte blood count< 100/mm^3. In the CSF, fungal meningitis produces no culture growth, reduces glucose levels, with elevated lymphocytes and protein. It is treated with amphotericin B, 5-flucytosine and antiretrovirals, with fluconazole prophylaxis.

13 – F

Multiple sclerosis is signalled by **oligoclonal IgG bands, relapsing-remitting** signs and symptoms, optic neuritis, raised CSF protein, no culture growth and L'Hermitte's sign (limb tingling on flexion of the neck, also seen with B12 deficiency and cervical spondylosis). Other EMQs may mention characteristic **delayed visual, auditory or somatosensory evoked potentials** on EEG, raised CSF lymphocyte count, antibodies to myelin oligodendrocyte glycoprotein and the **sunray sign** on sagittal gadolinium-enhanced MRI.

14 – H

JC papovavirus causes **progressive multifocal leucoencephalopathy**, an AIDS-defining illness, tending to occur with CD4 blood count <100/mm^3. Other features include ataxia, wasting, dementia, dysphonia, spasticity and sensory loss. MRI tends to show hypointense lesions on T1, while CSF produces no culture growth, with possible small increases in protein and lymphocyte level. Timely antiretroviral treatment prevents PML developing. Once it manifests, antiretrovirals can produce minor improvements.

15 – I

Ziehl-Neelsen stain of sputum or CSF detects acid-fast organsims such as mycobacterium **tuberculosis**. Other investigations for tuberculosis include chest x-rays, sputum cultures (require up to 12 weeks), Elispot, and HIV test. Normally, initial tuberculosis infection resolves in weeks. Post-primary tuberculosis results from subsequent immunocompromise, allowing the mycobacterium to escape from caseating granulomas at the **Ghon focus** (peripheral lesion, often at the lung or ileocaecal junction) and its **Ghon complex** (draining lymph nodes). Post-primary tuberculosis can reactivate in the lungs, infect other sites, or spread diffusely (miliary tuberculosis).

Tuberculous meningitis can be treated with a 12-month course of **R**ifampicin and **I**soniazid, combined with **P**yrazinamide and a fourth drug such as **E**thambutol for the first 2 months, (this can be remembered as **RIPE**) with vitamin B6 supplements (isoniazid reduces absorption) and possibly a course of dexamethasone to reduce CNS inflamation. Standard treatment of pulmonary tuberculosis is **RIPE**, with 2 months of RIPE and 4 subsequent months of RI alone. To ensure the treatment's completion, this may have to be given as Direct Observed Treatment. Drug-resistant variants would necessitate other regimens. Patients with suspected open pulmonary tuberculosis (i.e. sputum positive) should be isolated in negative pressure rooms until they have taken 2 weeks of effective anti-tuberculous treatment. On diagnosis, the consultant in communicable disease control should be notified, contact tracing and testing is mandatory as they may need full treatment, drug prophylaxis or vaccination.

The BCG vaccine has ~70% efficacy in the UK but is ineffective in tropical countries. 2 billion people worldwide are thought to be infected (mostly latent); it kills ~3m people per year, often in combination with HIV.

Further Information (Q. 11 – 15)

Meningitis types and CSF profiles

	Neutrophil count /mm³	Glucose mM	Lymphocyte Count /mm³	Protein g/L	Cell count /mm³	Appearance
Normal	0	2.8–4.2	<5	0.15-0.45	<5	clear
Bacterial	Very high can be >1000	<0.5*	can be raised	raised 1-5	Raised	turbid
TB	can be raised	<0.5*	raised	raised >1	Raised	filmy
Viral	can be raised	normal	raised	raised <1	Raised	clear
Fungal	can be raised	<0.5*	raised	raised	normal/ raised	often clear

*as proportion of blood levels

Acute disseminated encephalomyelitis (ADEM) typically follows viral infection or vaccination and causes acute immunopathologic demyelination, with rapid-onset UMN signs, fever, headache, cranial nerve palsies, seizures and ataxia. CSF protein and lymphocytes may be elevated; T2 MRI tends to show subcortical hyperintense white matter lesions. Neurosyphilis occurs years after infection and includes meningovascular (CVA and cranial nerve palsies), general paralysis of the insane (causing dementia), tabes dorsalis (dorsal column affected) and taboparesis (paresis and dorsal column damage) forms. Investigations include syphilis serology and STI screening. Procaine benzylpenicillin should ideally be started long before complications develop, alongside steroids to prevent the Jarisch-Herxheimer inflammatory reaction. Contact tracing is required. Contraindications to lumbar puncture include suspected raised intracranial pressure with risk of coning (CT scan can rule this out) clotting problems and lumbar sepsis. Causes of culture-negative meningitis include cancer, encephalitis, syphilis, subarachnoid haemorrhage, tuberculous/ non-bacterial/ partially treated bacterial infection, connective tissue disease and intrathecal drugs

---

16 – B

Angle closure glaucoma is suggested by **long-sightedness, haloes** and **nocturnal eye pain** (on pupil dilatation). Contact between the iris and cornea blocks drainage of the aqueous humour by the scleral sinuses and it may also feature nausea and visual field narrowing. Acute angle closure glaucoma is a medical emergency, intra-ocular pressure can be reduced by acetazolamide and pilocarpine (constricts the pupils, opening scleral sinus) before iridectomy surgery.

17 – D

An impaired corneal reflex can be caused by palsy of the ophthalmic (V1) division of the trigeminal nerve, which traverses the cavernous sinus. **Cavernous sinus thrombosis** usually results from bacterial sinus infection, requiring urgent antibiotic treatment. Her diplopia results from abducens (VI) palsy, other signs include oculomotor (III) and trochlear (IV) palsies (they all pass through the cavernous sinus), papilloedema, photophobia, retinal haemorrhages and blindness.

18 – C

Bacterial conjunctivitis is differentiated from anterior uveitis and acute angle closure glaucoma by **crusting** and intact acuity. Bacterial conjunctivitis is caused by staphylococci, streptococci and haemophilus and becomes bilateral due to the eye being rubbed.

19 – A

The positive **Talbot's test** is characteristic of iritis, occurring when eye pain increases on pupil constriction and convergence. **Bamboo spine** is pathognomic of ankylosing spondylitis, a form of seronegative arthritis. It may result in back pain, combined neck hyperextension, thoracic kyphosis and loss of lumbar lordosis, causing "question-mark posture". Features of ankylosing spondylitis can be remembered by "the 8 A's":
- **Anterior uveitis** (iris and ciliary body inflammation);
- **A**pical lung fibrosis;
- **A**ortic regurgitation;

- AV node block (varying degrees, due to fibrosis of the conduction system)
- Amyloidosis (can cause renal impairment);
- Atlanto-axial subluxation (risk of cord compression and quadriplegia)
- Achilles tendonitis;
- Axial arthritis (affecting spine and sacro-iliac joints).

Though keratitis is associated with ankylosing spondylitis, this diagnosis is less likely because there is no mention of white spots (formed by white blood cells) on the conjunctiva. While Sjogren's causes red eyes and is associated with arthropathy, it tends to be bilateral and cause dryness of epithelial surfaces in the mouth, eyes, parotid glands and sexual organs.

20 – J
Trachoma, caused by Chlamydia trachomatis, is the only option which affects the eyelashes, inverting them (entropion) and damaging the cornea. It is the commonest cause of blindness, with ~6 million cases annually and ~500 million current infections. It is treated with 8 weeks of daily tetracycline ointment, or 1 dose of azithromycin. The WHO developed the SAFE approach- surgery, antibiotics, facial cleanliness, environmental improvement.

Further Information (Q. 15 – 20)
Conjunctival haemorrhages, on inspection have a posterior limit visible beyond which the blood doesn't pass. The corneal surface and pupil are both normal and the condition is self-limiting. Subconjunctival haemorrhage displays no posterior limit, but again has a normal corneal surface and pupil. Graves' disease results from antibodies to the TSH receptor at the thyroid, which can cause propotosis, red eyes, periorbital swelling, lid lag, diplopia, papilloedema and hyperthyroid symptoms like goitre, weight loss, tremor, heat intolerance and exaggerated tendon reflexes. Infective keratitis is predisposed by contact lens misuse and malnutrition (particularly vitamin A deficiency). Corneal lesions stain green with fluorescein drops and are usually diagnosed by slit lamp examination followed by urgent same day referral, as complications include scarring and visual loss.

21 – D
The key word is **violaceous**, suggesting **dermatomyositis**. This can also cause distinctive lilac (heliotrope) papules on the knuckles, elbows and

knees (Gottren's sign). It may also feature lung fibrosis, and dysphagia. It is associated with cancer, particularly of the lungs, breast, gastrointestinal tract, breast and ovaries, in up to 10% of adult cases.

22 – B

LMN leg signs and **back pain** suggest **cauda equina syndrome**, due to nerve root compression. Other key features include perineal and buttock anaesthesia, bladder, bowel and sexual dysfunction. Spinal cord compression would cause UMN signs.

23 – G

The cue word is **pneumonia**. **Guillain-Barré syndrome** is an acute inflammatory polyradiculoneuropathy causing ascending, mostly transient LMN weakness and occurring after infection with bacteria like mycoplasma pneumoniae, campylobacter jejuni and the viruses HIV, influenza (including vaccine), CMV and Epstein-Barr. Complete paralysis may occur, and it can be fatal without respiratory support. Investigations include respiratory function, nerve conduction studies, HIV testing and serology (may be GM-1 antibody positive). The duration of symptoms can be shortened by intravenous immunoglobulin or plasma exchange.

24 – C

The **common peroneal nerve** encircles the head of the **fibula**; fracture here causes peroneal palsy. The peroneal nerve supplies the anterior compartment of the lower leg- including muscles required for ankle dorsiflexion (tibialis anterior, extensor digitorum) and eversion (peronei). The tibial nerve supplies the hamstrings (biceps femoris, semitendinosus and semimembranosus), muscles of the posterior compartment, required for ankle plantar flexion (e.g. gastrocnemius) and all muscle of the foot. Tibial palsy would cause limping, absent ankle jerk and absent plantar reflex, with numbness of the sole.

25 – F

Childhood onset suggests **Duchenne's muscular dystrophy** (prevalence ~1 per 4000 live male births) as opposed to Becker's. Gower's sign is the inability to stand up from the floor without the use of the arms. Becker's and Duchenne's are recessive X-linked progressive proximal dystrophies caused by dystrophin mutations. CK is likely to be raised, with characteristic fat infiltration on muscle biopsy (causing calf and deltoid pseudohypertrophy). Duchenne's muscular dystrophy causes disability, often necessitating wheelchair use by the patient's 2nd decade. The subsequent development of respiratory failure means average life expectancy ranges from 20 to 35. Becker's muscular dystrophy has an almost unreduced life expectancy, with the need for a wheelchair typically starting in the 5th decade.

Further Information (Q. 21 – 25)

Diabetic neuropathy is the commonest cause of autonomic neuropathy in the world and also affects the sensory and motor systems. Autonomic damage can have disparate effects such as erectile dysfunction, postural hypotension, constipation or diarrhoea, urine retention and is correlated with reduced life expectancy. Sensory neuropathy can cause numbness and pain from disorganised activation, typically in a glove-and stocking distal distribution. Microvascular complications such as retinopathy and neuropathy were shown to be prevented by tight glucose control (HbA1C< 7.5%) in the UKPDS (on type II diabetes) and DCCT (on type I) prospective cohort trials. Spinal cord compression can be caused by atlantoaxial subluxation, tumours, abscesses, disc prolapses, spondylosis and stenosis. Lesions affecting segments C3-5 compromise diaphragm motility and respiration. Compression of cord segment C8 may lead to LMN symptoms in the hands, with UMN symptoms in the legs. S3-4 compression causes perineal anaesthesia, loss of the anal reflex but normal motor function in the upper and lower limbs.

---

26 – I

The dissociated **loss of pain and temperature sensation** in a "**cape distribution**" and the **peripheral face** suggests **syringobulbia**, a presentation often alluded to in exams due to its involvement of several sensory-motor pathways. In the scenario, the syrinx (fluid-filled tube) extends upwards to the brainstem, combining **LMN signs** in the **arms** (C5-C8 distribution) by compressing anterior horn cells, **LMN cranial nerve palsies** (V, IX, X, XII) by disrupting brainstem nuclei and **UMN signs** in the **legs** by compressing the lateral corticospinal tract. Amyotrophy is loss of reflexes and atrophy. Dissociated sensory loss results from disruption of the **spinothalamic tract** as it passes close to the central canal, sparing the dorsal columns that carry vibroception, proprioception and fine touch. Pain and temperature sensation from the face is transmitted via the trigeminal (V) nucleus in the medulla and upper cervical spinal cord, with a **rostrocaudal** somatotopic "**onion-skin**" arrangement centred on the nose, as opposed to the mandibular, maxillary and ophthalmic dermatomes of the V nerve branches. Inferior V nucleus lesions affect the peripheral face-chin, scalp and ears, higher lesions affect the cheeks, nose and lips, while even higher lesions affect the teeth and pharynx. The trigeminal sensory nucleus for fine touch and the motor nucleus are found in the pons, while the trigeminal sensory nucleus for proprioception is found at the midbrain. Syringobulbia can also cause Horner's syndrome, LMN facial (VII) palsy and vestibulocochlear (VIII) palsy.

27 – E

Tongue fasciculations are virtually pathognomic of **motor neurone disease**, a rare (incidence 2-3/100 000/year) degenerative condition affecting the anterior horn cells, descending tracts and motor nuclei of the medulla, which can cause **mixed UMN** and **LMN** signs. Investigations include muscle biopsy, EMG and MRI of the neuro-axis to exclude differentials like multiple sclerosis and cervical spondylosis. Most people don't survive 5 years after diagnosis, though there are exceptions; in India, onset tends to be earlier with a more benign progression. Palliation includes muscle relaxants, physiotherapy and PEG feeding (preventing aspiration pneumonia). Riluzole, a glutamate antagonist, slightly increases life expectancy, suggesting damage due to excitotoxicity.

28 – J

Chvostek's sign is the main clue; specific to **hypocalcaemia**, it occurs when **gentle tapping under the ear** causes a **twitch on the same side of the face**. **Trousseau's sign**, also caused by **hypocalcaemia**, occurs when **blocking arterial flow** with a sphygmomanometer cuff to the upper arm, causes **metacarpophalangeal joint flexion, finger extension and thumb adduction**. The operation was a **thyroidectomy,** which can damage the neighbouring parathyroid gland, reducing parathyroid hormone (PTH) production to cause hypocalcaemia. Neuromuscular irritability results, with hypertonicity (e.g. carpopedal spasm) and exaggerated reflexes. Hypocalcaemia can also be caused by malabsorption, calcium or vitamin D deficiency, renal failure and hyperventilation.

29 – A

Anterior cerebral artery CVA damages the upper region of the primary motor cortex, affecting the **legs** more than the arms and face, while middle cerebral artery supplies the inferior motor cortex so a middle cerebral artery CVA affects the face and arms more than the legs. CVA's affecting the internal capsule or from carotid artery blockage may affect the legs, arms and face equally.

30 – H

Hashimoto's thyroiditis is a clue because it is an **autoimmune** condition associated with **pernicious anaemia**, which causes **B12 deficiency** and **subacute degeneration of the spinal cord**. Though hypothyroidism can cause confusion and dementia, it doesn't cause the UMN signs described. B12 deficiency causes peripheral neuropathy (LMN lesion) alongside dementia and spinal cord degeneration (UMN lesion), which can result in loss of knee and ankle reflexes, while the plantar reflex, served by more diffuse afferents, remains intact and displays the UMN Babinski sign. With regular vitamin B12 injections, much of the damage is reversible. Pernicious anaemia incurs an increased risk of gastric carcinoma. Other causes of B12 deficiency include malnutrition and terminal ileum disease. Some countries have mandatory folic acid supplementation of bread for prevention of neural tube birth defects. However, increased folic acid intake can mask macrocytosis in people with pernicious anaemia, increasing the likelihood of subacute degeneration of the spinal cord (co-supplementation with B12 would be no use because it would not be absorbed).

Further Information (Q. 26 – 30)

Although the question describes symptoms of bulbar palsy (LMN signs in cranial nerves IX, X and XII), the upper and lower limbs are also affected, making syringobulbia a better answer. Pseudobulbar palsy is an UMN lesion of the same cranial nerves, which may also display signs of frontal lobe damage such as emotional liability and UMN limb signs. Nerves IX, X and XII receive bilateral cortical input, thus UMN lesions involve bilateral damage.

	Gag reflex	Voice	Tongue	Jaw jerk
Pseudoglobular	Exaggerated	Spastic dysphonia	Hypertonic	Increased
Bulbar palsy	Reduced	Nasal	Fasciculation, Atrophy	Not present

Causes of pseudobulbar palsy include: motor neurone disease, CVA, multiple sclerosis. Causes of bulbar palsy include: motor neurone disease, myasthenia gravis, Guillain-Barré syndrome, syringobulbia.

31 – I
Focal signs are displayed, but the AIDS-defining cerebral **toxoplasmosis** is more likely than CVA due to the **fever, papilloedema, diarrhoea** and **weight loss**. In an immunocompromised person, cerebral abscesses form, causing focal signs, seizures, fever, chorioretinitis, confusion and headache with features of raised intracranial pressure.

32 – B
Tertian fever is the key phrase, virtually pathognomic of **malaria**, to which this person is vulnerable due to their implied **travel history**. Tertian or periodic fever spikes every third day, due to the parasite's breeding cycle. Investigations include Giemsa- stained thick and thin blood films for parasite counts, clotting screens, FBC, U&E, ABG, bicarbonate, glucose and lactate levels. Cerebral malaria has a mortality rate of ~20% and malaria kills 1-3 million people per year. Plasmodium falciparum is resistant to chloroquine; treatments include quinine, fansidar and artemether. Preventative measures include public health measures such as clearance of stagnant water breeding sites, insecticide-treated bed nets, avoiding exposure at dusk, long-sleeves and malaria prophylaxis tablets for tourists.

33 – C
CVA is suggested by the **focal signs** without features of infection. Incidence is ~1.5 per 1000 people per year in the UK and is the 3rd commonest cause of death behind cardiovascular disease and cancer. ~80% of CVA's are non-haemorrhagic, ~50% of these are due to atherosclerosis (large vessel disease), ~25% to lipohyalinosis (small vessel disease), ~20% due to cardiac emboli. Lipohyalinosis is due to hypertension causing fibrinoid necrosis at perforating vessels, and causes more limited signs than atherosclerotic CVA e.g. isolated sensory loss. ~10% of all CVA's are due to subarachnoid haemorrhage and ~10% to intracerebral haemorrhage. Risk factors for atherosclerosis include hypertension, smoking history, diabetes mellitus, high cholesterol, old age and family history. Early-onset CVA may be caused by fibromuscular dysplasia, an occlusive thickening of the tunica media, which can also affect renal vessels. Standard investigations include FBC, glucose, ESR, U&E, lipid profile, ECG, chest x-ray, CT head scan and Doppler ultrasound of the carotids. Treatment includes aspirin and dipyridamole (unless the CVA is haemorrhagic), statins, IV fluids, swallow assessment (may need to be nil-by mouth with nasogastric or PEG feeding to prevent aspiration pneumonia), glucose control, oxygen support, bed sore avoidance nursing and rehabilitative physiotherapy. Haemorrhagic CVA's may show improvement

on clot evacuation surgery. Hypertension is likely as a compensatory measure, treating this too early can further compromise cerebral blood supply. Thrombolysis can improve outcome of atherosclerotic CVA, if given within 3 hours of onset, but this requires CT to exclude haemorrhage. ~ 40% of patients make a full recovery and prognosis is better when treated in a stroke unit.

34 – H
Subdural haemorrhage is associated with **alcoholism** and old age. Subdural haemorrhages are venous and low-pressure, slowly accumulating between the dura mater and arachnoid mater to cause gradual cognitive deterioration, a differential of Alzheimer's. Foremost are features of mental slowing, drowsiness, unsteadiness and personality change. Signs of raised intracranial pressure, such as Cushing reflex (hypertension and bradycardia) develop early, while focal signs often emerge months later. Clot evacuation via burr holes can produce a complete recovery. Other causes of drowsiness to be considered in alcoholic patients include overdose, sepsis, hypoglycaemia and Wernicke-Korsakoff syndrome; hence there is a low threshold for initiation of vitamin infusions with glucose.

35 – D
The scenario describes the classical **lucid interval** which can occur with **extradural haemorrhage**. A haematoma accumulates rapidly between the skull and dura mater due to an arterial bleed. Intracranial pressure is initially compensated by CSF resorption and ventricle shrinkage, maintaining brain function. Subsequently, pressure rises and fatal brainstem coning can occur. Urgent haematoma evacuation is required following transfer to a neurological centre, where the bleeding artery can be ligated.

Further Information (Q. 31 – 35)
Transient ischaemic attacks cause symptoms lasting less than 24 hours, before regressing completely. They are most likely due to small clot emboli being expelled up the carotids to block cerebral vessels, which subsequently disperse. They may occur as harbingers of larger emboli, causing permanent ischaemic damage. Arrhythmias and artificial heart valve replacements predispose to clot formation, often requiring long-term anticoagulant therapy with warfarin. Carotid artery stenosis also contributes and, if narrowed by 70% or more on Doppler ultrasound, carotid endarterectomy surgery is indicated.

36 – C

Even without the classic non-blanching rash, **meningococcal septicaemia** may still be present and is suggested by the leg pain, peripheral coolness, fever and vomiting without diarrhoea.

37 – A

Brown-Séquard syndrome is caused by lesions affecting half the transverse surface of the spinal cord. This can result from **Human T-lymphotrophic virus-1** (HTLV-1), a sexually and vertically transmitted infection widespread in Africa, the Caribbean, Japan, South America and the southern USA. Unilateral UMN signs result, with dissociated loss of pain and temperature sensation contralaterally (spinothalamic tract damaged which decussates just above its level of entry), while fine touch, proprioception and vibroception are lost ipsilaterally (dorsal columns damaged which decussate at the medulla) below the lesion.

38 – I

Her **Burmese** origins are a clue, because **measles vaccination** does not have full coverage there. She has **subacute sclerosing panencephalitis**, a rare and incurable delayed complication of measles infection in early life, causing progressive brain damage, seizures, and UMN signs. Commoner clinical features of measles include fever, cough, Koplik's spots (grey irregular lesions of the mouth), and rash, with complications of bacterial pneumonia, gastroenteritis and myocarditis more likely in malnourished children.

39 – E

Lightning pains (stabbing, irregular, brief and localised) suggest **tabes dorsalis**; impaired dorsal column function caused by neurosyphilis. The loss of reflexes, stamping gait and ataxia are caused by reduced sensory input- to feel the floor, they need to exert more force. There may also be Charcot joints (advanced damage due to loss of pain input), ptosis and Argyll Robertson pupils. The Argyll-Robertson pupil demonstrates accommodation but not a direct light response (light-near dissociation). Tying it to neurosyphilis (one of its causes) and the fact that it "accommodates but does not react", some people remember it as "the prostitute's pupil".

 Another way of remembering it would be **A**rgyll **R**obertson **P**upil shortened to **ARP** forwards, **PRA** backwards- **A**ccommodation

Response Present, Pupillary Response Absent. It is generally caused by lesions around the aqueduct of Sylvius in the midbrain.

40 – F

This is **taboparesis**, caused by congenital syphilis infection, combining signs of tabes dorsalis and "generalised paralysis of the insane. In the UK, screening for syphilis antibodies is standard for pregnant women, alongside antibodies to other pathogens such as HIV, hepatitis B and rubella.

Further Information (Q. 36 – 40)

Tuberculomas are chronic caseating granulomas containing mycobacteria. AIDS-defining CNS conditions, each of which tend to develop with CD4 count <100/mm^3, include progressive multifocal leucoencephalopathy, cerebral toxoplasmosis, cytomegalovirus (CMV) retinitis, CMV encephalitis, CMV radiculopathy, CNS non-Hodgkin's lymphoma, and HIV encephalopathy. Highly active antiretroviral therapy (HAART) prevents AIDS developing, if started early enough. A typical regimen would be 2 nucleoside reverse transcriptase inhibitors (e.g. tenofovir and emtricitabine) and a boosted protease inhibitor (e.g. lopinavir and ritonavir).

By the end of 2007, UNAIDS/WHO estimated there were ~33 million people living with HIV and AIDS worldwide, including ~22 million in sub-Saharan Africa. During 2007, ~2.7 million (including ~0.37 million children) were estimated to have been infected, while ~2 million (including ~0.27 million children) died. Approximately 25 million people have died of AIDS-related illnesses so far. Adult HIV prevalence exceeds 15% in countries such as South Africa, Zimbabwe, Namibia, Botswana and Lesotho (UNAIDS 2007). In Brazil, the availability of free generic antiretroviral therapy since 1996, produced despite opposition from drugs multinationals, is estimated to have halved HIV-related deaths between 1996 and 1999 and saved more than $2 billion in treatment costs over 10 years (Teixeira et al 2003). Ugandan prevention initiatives included grass roots HIV support groups, increasing condom use and behaviour change. Combined with a high death rate, Ugandan adult HIV prevalence fell from 15% in the early 90s to 5.4% in 2007. In 2007, the WHO fund to fight AIDS, tuberculosis and malaria delivered antiretroviral treatment to almost 3 million HIV positive people in developing countries (reaching 80% coverage in Argentina, Brazil, Chile, Cuba and Namibia), out of ~9.7 million that needed it.

41 – B
These are **dopa-decarboxylase inhibitors,** such as **benserazide.** These reduce the peripheral breakdown of levodopa, allowing it to cross the blood brain barrier.

42 – I
Selegiline is a monoamine oxidase B inhibitor. This enzyme breaks down dopamine; inhibiting it increases dopamine levels. Bromocriptine, pergolide and ropinerole are dopamine agonists, which can be used before levodopa to treat Parkinson's. Benserazide is an enzyme inhibitor given alongside levodopa.

43 – A
Apomorphine is a dopamine agonist which can cause nausea, for which reason it may be given alongside **domperidone,** which blocks dopamine action at the chemoreceptor trigger zone.

44 – C
Benzhexol is an antimuscarinic drug, which can have the central side-effect of confusion.

45 – B
Benserazide is a dopa-decarboxylase inhibitor given alongside levodopa in **co-beneldopa.**

Further Information (Q. 41 – 45)
Parkinson's disease is an idiopathic condition caused by damage to the basal ganglia, specifically the substantia nigra pars compacta dopamine-releasing neurones in the midbrain, with presence of Lewy bodies on microscopy. It has a prevalence of ~0.2% in the general population, with incidence ~20 per 100,000 per year, tending to affect elderly people. Treatment includes levodopa and a dopa-decarboxylase inhibitor to prevent peripheral conversion to dopamine.

Dopamine is less lipophilic than levodopa, hence cannot cross the blood brain barrier but causes peripheral effects such as labile hypertension, dizziness and tachyarrhythmias when converted to noradrenaline and emesis by activating the chemoreceptor trigger zone. Levodopa only works for a limited time before on-off effects set in. Other treatments include amantadine, selegiline, entacapone (prevents the methylation of dopamine, reducing on-off effects) and dopamine agonists.

Neurosurgical approaches include thalamotomy and pallidotomy. Other avenues of research are electrode implants and stem cell transplants to replace dopamergic substantia nigra. Bromocriptine is a dopamine agonist used to reduce prolactin secretion by the anterior pituitary gland in galactorrhoea.

---

46 – J
The mention of **acute leukaemia** suggests a drug side-effect as the cause. Vinca alkaloids are used in chemotherapy combinations for the treatment of acute leukaemias and lymphomas and cause **neurotoxicity**. **Vincristine** is for intravenous use only; deaths have been caused by accidental intrathecal injection. Chlorambucil is a chemotherapeutic alkylating drug used to treat chronic lymphocytic leukaemia; its main side effect is bone marrow suppression and it does not cause neuropathy.

47 – D
Her **pregnancy** is relevant because it, along with obesity, predisposes to **meralgia paraesthetica** in which the lateral cutaneous nerve of the thigh is trapped under the inguinal ligament.

48 – A
These areas are all innervated by cervical nerve roots, indicating **cervical rib syndrome**. This condition is explained by some as stemming from fibrous bands growing from C7's transverse process to compress the lower brachial plexus roots at C8 and T1, leading to wasting and weakness of the small muscles of the hand, with pain and numbness in the C8 and T1 distribution. Horner's syndrome can develop and with an obstructed subclavian artery, blood pressure is unequal in each arm.

49 – G
The muscles of the **forearm's extensor compartment**, affected here, are innervated by the **radial nerve**. Sleeping with an arm resting over a chair compresses the radial nerve in the spiral groove on the medial humerus, causing **"Saturday night palsy"**. **Intact triceps jerk indicates intact radial nerve above the spiral groove**. Traumatic radial nerve palsy can

also be caused by ill-fitting crutches. Recovery is normally spontaneous within months.

50 – E

Hypopigmented anaesthetic skin lesions are pathognomic of **leprosy**, which is a more specific answer than the mononeuritis multiplex it is causing in the scenario. Leprosy is the commonest cause of mononeuritis multiplex worldwide, affecting ~3 million people, and is due to the acid-fast mycobacterium leprae. Lepromatous leprosy is the most severe form, occurring with dysfunctional cell-mediated immunity; lesions are diffuse and impaired nociception causes progressive injuries. Diagnosis is clinical or on obtaining skin and nasal mucosa swabs of acid-fast bacteria. Treatment options include a 2-year regimen of once-monthly rifampicin and clofazamine depots, plus daily clofazamine and dapsone maintenance, often directly observed to ensure concordance.

Further Information (Q. 46 – 50)

Peripheral neuropathy has numerous causes, such as paraneoplastic phenomenon, diabetes, uraemia and alcoholism. Charcot-Marie-Tooth is hereditary motor-sensory neuropathy causing distal muscle atrophy ("inverted champagne bottle legs"), thickened nerves and absent reflexes. Ulnar palsy can be caused by pressure at the elbow, compressing the nerve at the olecranon groove. Tuberculosis treatment with isoniazid can cause peripheral neuropathy; prophylactic pyridoxine (vitamin B6) is given to prevent this.

---

51 – B

The scenario suggests **bacterial meningitis**, a clinical emergency. Delaying antibiotics to await blood results can be fatal. GP's tend to carry benzylpenicillin on house visits, for intramuscular injection in suspected cases of bacterial meningitis while awaiting the ambulance. Benzylpenicillin is effective against most strains of streptococcus pneumonia and neisseria meningitidis in the UK (resistance is higher in South Africa, Spain and USA) but not haemophilus. Cefotaxime is given IV and is effective against neisseria, streptococcus and haemophilus. Dexamethasone is given early in meningitis to reduce the risk of long-term complications such as deafness. It is avoided in septicaemic meningitis, confirmed meningococcal infection or with immunocompromised patients.

52 – E
The positive **Indian ink** stain indicates the fungus **Cryptococcus**, which is causing AIDS-defining cryptococcal meningitis.

53 – C
These features all suggest **herpes simplex encephalitis**, which is treated with intravenous aciclovir.

54 – G
Cases of **meningococcal** infection require **public health notification**; contacts must be traced and given antibacterial prophylaxis. Rifampicin is the standard prophylactic treatment but as a P450 enzyme inducer, it disrupts the efficacy of oral contraceptives, in which case **ciprofloxacin** is preferred.

55 – J
This suggests the AIDS-defining illness **cerebral toxoplasmosis**, causing a cerebral abscess. Folinic acid is required because pyrimethamine reduces folate absorption. Mortality is ~70% and steroids may also be needed to reduce oedema. Though cerebral toxoplasmosis is an AIDS-defining illness, HIV-positive patients can suffer brain abscesses from other causes such as staphylococcus or tuberculosis. However, **J** is the only listed option appropriate for treatment of a brain abscess.

Causes of ring-enhancing lesions can be remembered by the mnemonic **MAGIC DR** – **M**etastases, **A**bscesses, **G**lioma and other primary brain tumours, **I**nfarction, **C**ontusion, **D**emyelination, **R**esolving haematoma.

Further Information (Q. 51 – 55)
Cefotaxime is a cephalosporin antibiotic that can only be given intravenously or intramuscularly. Erythromycin is a macrolide, suitable for people allergic to penicillin and used in the treatment of mycoplasma or chlamydia pneumonia. Co-trimoxazole is a mixture of sulphamethoxazole and trimethoprim used for the treatment and prophylaxis of pneumocystis jiroveci fungal pneumonia, an AIDS-defining condition. It is also used in prophylaxis of toxoplasmosis infection. Where antiretroviral programmes are not available, prophylaxis with co-trimoxazole can extend the lifespan of HIV-positive patients; the WHO recommends it for children born of mothers suspected to be HIV-positive.

56 – H

She has partial seizures with no secondary generalisation; first-line treatments include **lamotrigine**, sodium valproate, carbamazepine, oxcarbazepine and topiramate (NICE 2004). Valproate may worsen polycystic ovarian syndrome and is a p450 enzyme inhibitor, while carbamazepine is a p450 inducer, therefore Option H is the best choice.

57 – H

The scenario suggests **absence seizures** (AKA petit mal), a form of **generalised epilepsy**. First-line treatments of childhood absence seizures include sodium valproate, ethosuximide and **lamotrigine** (NICE 2004), of which the latter is considered safest in pregnancy.

Epilepsy medication can **impair folic acid absorption**, increasing the risk of **neural tube defects** - 0.2-0.5% in the general population, 1-2% when taking valproate and 1% or less with **carbamazepine**; there is less data on newer drugs. Not taking medication could harm the foetus by increasing the risk of a generalised seizure and miscarriage.

All epileptic women attempting to become pregnant while on medication require specialist advice and should take 5mg daily folic acid supplements to reduce the risk of neural tube defects.

Carbamazepine, gabapentin, oxcarbazepine, tiagabine and vigabatrin can worsen absence seizures.

58 – H

The scenario is characteristic of **juvenile myoclonic epilepsy**, a form of **generalised seizure**. First-line treatments include sodium valproate and **lamotrigine** (NICE 2004); the former is contraindicated by her active liver disease (BNF). Lamotrigine therapy can cause rashes and entails a small risk of serious reactions like Stevens-Johnson syndrome and toxic epidermal necrolysis, particularly in children, about which warnings should be given before prescribing. Carbamazepine, oxcarbazepine, phenytoin, tiagabine and vigabatrin can worsen juvenile myoclonic epilepsy.

59 – J

The history of **bone marrow depression** is relevant because it contraindicates carbamazepine and is a caution against prescribing lamotrigine, both first-line treatments for the suggested childhood tonic-clonic seizure (AKA grand mal), alongside **sodium valproate** and topiramate (NICE

2004). Tiagabine and vigabatrin are to be avoided in myoclonic epilepsy as they can worsen the condition.

60 – B

The scenario suggests progression to **status epilepticus**, a seizure or repeated seizures without recovery lasting longer than **30 minutes**; in ~50% of cases there is no prior history of seizures. This can be fatal, though conversely ~25% of cases of apparent cases are believed to be pseudostatus (non-epileptic attack), risking iatrogenic harm.

The patient should be placed in the recovery position if possible; intubation may be required to maintain an airway. It is aimed to stop the seizures within 20 minutes, first by **IV phenytoin**. If IV access is not possible, diazepam or paraldehyde can be given rectally, or if seizures continue other IV options include phenobarbitone and fosphenytoin.

Failure to respond may raise suspicions of pseudostatus. Prolonged genuine convulsions necessitate anaesthetic induction with thiopentone or propofol, followed by muscle paralysis and ventilation, with EEG seizure monitoring.

Further Information (Q. 56 – 60)
Both lamotrigine and sodium valproate are first-line treatments of tonic-clonic, childhood and juvenile absence epilepsy, myoclonic, tonic, atonic and partial seizures (i.e. all forms), while carbamazepine is first-line for tonic-clonic and partial seizures (NICE 2004). Carbamazepine is a liver p450 enzyme inducer (increases drug metabolism including oral contraceptive) while valproate is a p450 inhibitor. Carbamazepine plasma levels can be monitored during treatment, while valproate's are not because they are not related to its efficacy.

Newer first-line drugs are available, but as they have been available for a shorter time, their side-effects (particularly on pregnant women, who are never involved in drug trials) are less known. Phenytoin works against all forms of epilepsy apart from absence seizures, but is no longer first-line due to its side-effects of gum hyperplasia, facial coarsening, acne, hirstutism and fetal hydantoin syndrome (cleft lip, neural tube defects, congenital heart defects).

Clobazam and clonazepam are second-line therapies for several types of epilepsy. Gabapentin is a second-line treatment for partial seizures.

Further information (Q. 61 – 65)

Cranial nerve and skull exit point	Causes of lesions
I: Olfactory **Cribriform plate**	Increasing age, upper respiratory tract infection, smoking, trauma, meningioma.
II: Optic **Optic foramen**	Maculopathy, ischaemia, optic/ retrobulbar neuritis, retinoblastoma, nerve/ chiasm/ tract compression.
III: Oculomotor **Superior orbital fissure**	Aneurysm of posterior communicating artery, midbrain tumour, brainstem CVA (e.g. lateral medullary syndrome), cavernous sinus thrombosis/ tumour/ aneurysm. III sympathetic lesion alone: syringobulbia, lung cancer.
IV: Trochlear **Superior orbital fissure**	Cavernous sinus thrombosis/ tumour/ aneurysm/ vascular.
V: Trigeminal **Ophthalmic nerve (V1- superior orbital fissure), Maxillary nerve (V2- foramen rotundum). Mandibular nerve (V3- foramen ovale)**	Multiple sclerosis, CVA (e.g. lateral medullary syndrome, pontine CVA), cerebellopontine angle tumours (e.g. acoustic neuroma), syringobulbia, chronic meningitis, thrombosis/ tumour/ aneurysm of cavernous or inferior petrosal sinus.
VI: Abducens **Superior orbital fissure**	Raised intracranial pressure, trauma, pontine glioma/CVA, diabetes mellitus, Wernicke's encephalopathy, thrombosis/ tumour/ aneurysm of cavernous, lateral /inferior petrosal sinus.
VII: Facial **Stylomastoid foramen**	**UMN:** Frontal lobe CVA/ tumour. **LMN:** pontine CVA, cerebellopontine angle tumours (e.g. acoustic neuroma), idiopathic (Bell's), Varicella Zoster (Ramsay-Hunt), syringobulbia, sarcoidosis, Guillain-Barré syndrome (GBS), lateral sinus thrombosis/ tumour/ aneurysm, glomus tumour.
VIII: Vestibulocochlear **Internal acoustic meatus**	Conductive: otosclerosis, wax, otitis media. Sensorineural: Ototoxic drugs, trauma, infection, cerebellopontine angle tumours (e.g acoustic neuroma), brainstem CVA (e.g. lateral medullary syndrome). Vestibular syndromes: labyrinthitis, Meniere's disease.
IX: Glossopharyngeal **Jugular foramen**	GBS, motor neurone disease, brainstem CVA (e.g. lateral medullary syndrome), syringobulbia, jugular foramen lesion, MS.
X: Vagus **Jugular foramen**	**UMN:** motor neurone disease, MS, CVA. **LMN:** motor neurone disease, syringobulbia, GBS ,brainstem CVA (e.g. lateral medullary syndrome), jugular foramen lesion.
XI: Accessory **Jugular foramen**	Trauma, polio, syringomyelia, jugular foramen lesion.
XII: Hypoglossal **Hypoglossal canal**	**UMN:** Motor neurone disease, CVA, MS, **LMN:** GBS, motor neurone disease, syringobulbia.

Lesion signs
Anosmia, reduced taste.
Loss of sight, disc swelling, retinopathy, colour blindness, field defects, relative afferent pupillary defect, Argyll-Robertson pupil, impaired accommodation reflex.
Dilated unreactive pupil, ptosis, pupil pointing down and out, diplopia, Horner's syndrome, impaired accommodation reflex. Fixed dilatation with cerebral mass.
Cannot look down when eye adducted, diplopia.
UMN: weakness and exaggerated jaw jerk if lesion bilateral. **LMN**: Weakness and wasting of muscles of mastication. **Sensory**: loss of facial sensation and corneal reflex.
Convergent strabismus, nystagmus, diplopia.
UMN: contralateral facial weakness, occipitofrontalis spared, corneal reflex intact **LMN**: ipsilateral facial wasting and weakness, no sparing, Bell's phenomenon, dry eyes, corneal ulceration, external auditory meatus ulceration (Ramsay- Hunt) **Both**: loss of taste, hyperacusis, dry mouth, dysarthria, smoothing of nasolabial groove.
Conductive loss: Rinné negative, Weber test louder on affected side. Sensorineural loss: Weber test louder on unaffected side. Vestibular: wide-based gait, vomiting, nystagmus away from side of lesion. Romberg positive.
Reduced posterior palate sensation, weak gag reflex.
UMN: Exaggerated gag reflex, nasal high-pitched voice, possible emotional lability, UMN signs elsewhere. **LMN**: Weak gag reflex, hoarse/ nasal voice. **Both**: dysphagia, aspiration, regurgitation. Unilateral: uvula deviates towards unaffected side.
Weakness and wasting of trapezius and sternocleidomastoid muscles.
UMN: slowly moving, small tongue. **LMN**: tongue fasciculations, deviates towards affected side.

61 – E

Right accessory nerve (XI) supplies the trapezius and sternocleidomastoid, allowing rotation of the head to the opposite side.

62 – C

Left hypoglossal (XII nerve) causes the tongue to deviate towards the side of the lesion

63 – G

Facial weakness with **intact occipitofrontalis** function suggests **UMN facial nerve (VII) palsy**, as it has bilateral UMN innervation, unlike muscles lower down in the face. Bilateral frontal CVA could cause bilateral UMN VII signs with possible emotional lability.

64 – A

This is a **relative afferent pupillary defect**, (AKA Marcus-Gunn pupil) and is due to **unilateral optic nerve (II) damage.**

65 – I

The combination of **trigeminal (V), facial (VII)** and **vestibulocochlear (VIII)** cranial nerve palsy suggests **cerebellopontine angle tumour** (e.g. acoustic neuroma), due to the location of their nuclei in the brainstem.

---

66 – H

Mention of a **long flight** suggests **deep vein thrombosis**. A clot has passed from the venous to the arterial system via a septal defect (**paradoxical embolus**) to cause a CVA. These often manifest initially as flaccid weakness, developing over hours into spastic paresis, the classic features of an upper motor neurone injury. Small atrial septal defects may be detectable as right ventricular enlargement, with fixed splitting of the second heart sound on inspiration and diastolic tricuspid murmur due to increased bloodflow.

67 – J

The car crash resulted in a ruptured spleen, necessitating a **splenectomy**, causing **increased vulnerability to coated bacteria** like Haemophilus, Neisseria and Streptococcus. Annual vaccination to these bacteria and influenza is recommended, alongside daily phenoxymethylpenicillin antibiotic prophylaxis for 2 years or until they are 16 (whichever is longer) and carrying paramedic warning cards - if she develops even a minor infection, it is treated seriously.

68 – B

This is suggestive of **multiple sclerosis**, with initial presentation of optic neuritis. Risk of multiple sclerosis is higher in those who reached puberty in areas with **greater displacement north or south** from the equator, which is thought to relate to post-viral immunopathology. However, the noted "hot spot" of Orkney (0.12% prevalence compared to 0.04% in England and 0.001% below 30° North) has been attributed to genetic relic groups.

69 – G

This suggests mild **cerebral palsy**, mostly caused by brain damage in utero and predisposed by **prematurity**, defined as delivery before 36 weeks gestation. This also predisposes to autism, perinatal infection, birth defects, deafness, learning disabilities and visual impairment. Forms of cerebral palsy include infantile hemiparesis, congenital ataxia, spastic diplegia and athetoid.

70 – E

This describes movement characteristic of **Huntington's chorea**, alongside disinhibition from progressive subcortical dementia. It is a currently incurable degenerative condition of prevalence ~5 per 100,000, **inherited in autosomal dominant fashion**. Onset is mainly in middle age, though more CAG base repeats cause childhood disease; disability and death result within 10-20 years. Phenothiazines and tetrabenazine may help reduce abnormal movements. Offspring of people with Huntington's have a 50% chance of developing it; genetic counselling is available, though some may wish not to know. Other causes of choreiform movements include hyperthyroidism, benign hereditary chorea and Sydenham's chorea, hypocalcaemia, antipsychotic and anticonvulsant medication.

Further Information (Q. 66 – 70)

Cocaine use causes extreme hypertension, predisposing to atherosclerotic and haemorrhagic CVA's. Polycystic kidney disease is associated with berry aneurysms, predisposing to subarachnoid haemorrhage. Sickle cell disease occurs predominantly amongst people of African descent and is caused by a homozygous recessive mutation, with production of HbSS haemoglobin. Infection, cold weather, dehydration and pregnancy can increase blood viscosity and reduce oxygen concentration, causing HbSS to polymerise, blocking blood vessels, resulting in painful ischaemic self-promulgating sickling attacks, causing CVA, osteomyelitis, myocardial infarcts, aplastic crises, gangrene, priapism, renal papillary necrosis, acute chest syndrome and splenic dysfunction. Acute treatment includes opiate analgesia, rehydration, respiratory support, bronchodilators and antibiotics. Longer-term measures include vaccination against coated bacteria and influenza, parental education, genetic counselling, respiratory physiotherapy and hydroxyurea to increase the proportion of fetal haemoglobin, HbF, which does not sickle.

Poverty was described by Gandhi as "the greatest violence of all". According to the National Office for Statistics, within England and Wales (2002-2005), life expectancy for people in socio-economic class I (higher managerial and professional occupations) was 6.5 years greater than in class V (unskilled manual labour or unemployed), with an overall average of 79 years and infant mortality of 5 per 1000 (UNICEF 2007). Life expectancy in Angola, a country vastly rich in natural resources, is 42, with an infant mortality of 116 per 1000 (UNICEF 2007). In the UK, all diseases become more prevalent in passing from socio-economic class I to V, with exceptions including anorexia nervosa, bulimia nervosa, breast cancer, eczema, glandular fever, Hodgkin's disease of early adulthood, malignant melanoma and recessive conditions such as haemophilia in aristocratic dynasties.

71 – D
In addition, **Huntington's** causes neuronal loss at the corpus striatum.

72 – B
The **cerebellum** is responsible for fine coordination; **essential tremor** is an autosomal dominant condition featuring postural (during action) hand tremor exacerbated by anxiety and beta adrenergic agonists (e.g. salbutamol). It has been attributed to defects in the cerebellum and thalamus (Louis et al 2006). Tremor may spread to the head and trunk, worsening with age. Essential tremor is a differential of Parkinson's as the latter condition can also produce a postural tremor, in addition to the classical resting tremor. Treatment is often unnecessary, but symptoms are improved by small amounts of alcohol and beta blockers.

73 – C
Hemiballismus is jerky wild movements affecting one side of the body, caused by contralateral **subthalamic nucleus CVA.**

74 – E
These are called **Lewy bodies; Parkinson's** occurs with destruction of 80% or more of substantia nigra pars compacta cells.

75 – I
These are **Kayser-Fleischer rings**, pathognomic of **Wilson's disease**, due to **copper deposition** at the basal ganglia, liver and cornea, with childhood onset. Caeruloplasmin binds 90% of plasma copper; deficiency leads to more free copper ions, levels should be tested in children with akinetic-rigid symptoms or liver cirrhosis. Treatment is by the copper-chelating agent penicillamine without which cortical damage and learning difficulties result.

Further Information (Q. 71 – 75)
Primary torsion dystonia is a rare autosomal dominant, progressive condition featuring uncontrolled muscle contraction disrupting posture and gait. By the 4th decade, all four limbs are affected, though cognition remains intact. Sydenham's chorea can occur after rheumatic fever, caused by group A beta-haemolytic streptococcal infection in childhood. Recovery tends to occur spontaneously and gradually over months. Rheumatic fever can also cause acute carditis (with mitral or aortic regurgitation, flitting arthralgia, erythema marginatum and subcutaneous nodules) with long-term complications of aortic or mitral stenosis. It is treated with aspirin and phenoxymethylpenicillin, with antibiotic prophylaxis required for surgery and dental work to prevent infectious endocarditis.

76 – J
Six or more **"cafe-au-lait"** macules are found with adult Type 1 neurofibromatosis, alongside axillary and inguinal freckles and iris hamartomas (Lisch nodules). This autosomal dominant condition (~4 per 10 000 prevalence) causes myelin nerve sheath growths. It may also feature optic glioma, renal artery stenosis (causing secondary hypertension), learning disabilities and bone lesions.

77 – E
Depression is key because hyponatremia is a rare side-effect of specific serotonin reuptake inhibitor antidepressants.

78 – H
His **Spanish** nationality is relevant because the parasite Taenia Solium, which causes neurocysticercosis, is endemic in Spain, Eastern Europe, Africa, Asia and Latin America, causing a significant proportion of chronic epilepsy. Parasitic ova form brain cysts that degenerate to leave gliosis, calcification and inflammation, leading to seizures and neurological deficit. Treatment includes anti-epileptic medication, analgesia, corticosteroids, mannitol to control intracranial hypertension and anti-helmithic agents like albendazole. Surgery may be required for complicated cases.

79 – B
This is type of hallucination is encountered during **alcohol withdrawal**, which can lead to convulsions in **delirium tremens**.

80 – A
Causes of **DIC** include Gram-negative septicaemia (as in this case), burns, malignancy, trauma, mismatched transfusions and placental abruption. Clotting is extensive, blocking blood vessels, exhausting clotting factors and causing heavy bleeding.

Further Information (Q. 76 – 80)
Seizure is a normal response to brain insults including anoxia, electrolyte irregularities, space-occupying lesions, drug withdrawal, haemorrhage, fever and hypoglycaemia. Epilepsy is diagnosed after at least 2 seizures and most cases are idiopathic i.e. occurring in the absence of structural brain damage.

---

81 – A
Acoustic neuroma is a tumour of the vestibulocochlear (VIII) cranial nerve's Schwann cells. This requires neurosurgical intervention, which also risk damaging the trigeminal (V) and facial nerve (VII) as they are adjacent at the cerebellopontine angle.

82 – C
A mass in the **fourth ventricle** of a child suggests **ependymoma**, the 2nd commonest malignant brain tumour of childhood after medulloblastoma.

83 – D
Glioblastoma multiforme is the **most malignant** type of astocytoma, affecting adults in the frontal, parietal and temporal lobes.

84 – I
Pituitary adenomas cause **bitemporal hemianopia** when they compress the **optic chiasm**. The case described is causing acromegaly, leading to carpal tunnel syndrome and secondary diabetes due to excessive growth hormone (GH) release, other effects of which include organomegaly, obstructive sleep apnoea, proximal muscle weakness and gigantism if secretion starts before puberty. The oral glucose tolerance test involves ingestion of 75g glucose solution, which should normally reduce GH levels. Treatment is via transphenoidal surgery or external beam radiotherapy.

 Anterior pituitary hormones can be remembered by the mnemonic **GP SAT-** **G**rowth hormone, **P**rolactin, **S**ex hormones (LH and FSH), **A**CTH, **T**SH.

85 – J
The white colouration is called **leukocoria** and occurs with **retinoblastoma**, a highly malignant, inheritable childhood cancer of the retina (prevalence ~1 per 20 000). Retinoblastoma can be bilateral (more likely in the inherited form), causing strabismus, impaired vision, red and painful eyes, the cancer spreading from to the spinal cord and brain. Treatment options include enucleation (removal of eye and optic nerve), intrathecal chemotherapy and radiotherapy. Early diagnosis and treatment reduces mortality below 10%, but it is fatal without intervention. Survivors of retinoblastoma are at increased risk of osteosarcoma and melanoma.

Further Information (Q. 81 – 85)
Meningiomas (~20% of primary tumours) are benign tumours of the dura mater. Astrocytomas and oligodendrogliomas are types of glioma (~50% of primary brain tumours), tumours of varying malignancy originating from neuroglia. Oligodendrogliomas are slow-growing tumours of the brain's myelinating cells, occurring in adults, most commonly in the frontal lobe. Medulloblastoma develops from embryonic cerebellar tissue and is the

commonest malignant tumour of childhood. CNS lymphoma is an AIDS-defining aggressive B-cell neoplasm caused by Epstein-Barr virus, but can also present without HIV.

86 – B

Dementia with early development of **urinary incontinence** and **gait problems** suggests **colloid cyst** or normal-pressure hydrocephalus (occurs in the elderly). Colloid cysts are congenital, forming in the third ventricle to cause obstructing hydrocephalus with presentation mostly in adulthood. Dim vision and features of elevated intracranial pressure may also occur, with treatment by insertion of CSF shunts draining to the peritoneal space, or surgical excision.

87 – E

The key features are his **labile mood, loss of semantic knowledge** and **primitive reflex**, which suggest frontal lobe involvement, as opposed to the more diffuse pattern of advanced Alzheimer's. Semantic dementia is a **frontotemporal dementia** subtype, affecting conceptual knowledge early on.

88 – I

Lewy body dementia, the 3rd commonest form, features **Parkinsonian** symptoms, due to inclusion bodies at the cortex and basal ganglia. Though Parkinson's is not a form of dementia per se, dementia does occur more frequently with Parkinson's and may be of the Alzheimer's or Lewy-body type. Visual hallucinations may occur but antipsychotics are not recommended, as these worsen extrapyramidal symptoms and increase mortality.

89 – H

Smoking is a risk factor for **atherosclerosis** and **multiple-infarct dementia**, the 2nd commonest form. This tends to cause a stepwise progressive worsening of cognitive function with each minor CVA and possible UMN signs. There may be a history of TIA or a source of arterial clots such as atrial fibrillation, heart valve disease or carotid stenosis.

90 – A

These features, particularly **lucid intervals**, suggest severe **Alzheimer's**, the commonest form of dementia.

Further Information (Q. 86 – 90)

Creutzfeldt-Jakob disease is a rare spongiform encephalopathy recognised in original and new variant forms, causing dementia after a prolonged latent period. The new variant form is contracted by consuming beef from cows infected by bovine spongiform encephalopathy, containing prions which disrupt normal protein structure. It may also be transmitted by surgical instruments (even after heat treatment), blood transfusions and organ transplants. Folate deficiency causes cognitive impairment and results from a diet lacking green vegetables, pregnancy (increased intake by conceptus), haemolysis, tropical sprue, coeliac disease and drug side-effects (e.g. anti-epileptics). On investigation, macrocytic anaemia, megaloblastic bone marrow biopsy and low serum folate are likely. HIV encephalopathy is an AIDS-defining condition featuring subcortical dementia, tending to occur with CD4 count <200/mm³. Without antiretrovirals, 15-20% of HIV positive individuals develop it; antiretrovirals with high CSF penetration, such as zidovudine, lamivudine, indinavir and nevirapine are recommended, which may lead to partial cognitive improvement.

91 – D

The **grey spots** are key, termed **drusen** and suggestive of senile **macular degeneration**, presenting with gradual loss of central vision. Patients are therefore unable to recognise distant objects, but as peripheral vision remains, will usually be able to navigate. Treatment includes the non-licensed use of the anti-angiogenic monoclonal antibody bevacizumab, normally prescribed for bowel cancer

92 – C

Advanced **hypertensive retinopathy** can cause **disc swelling**, enlarging the area without photoreceptors where the optic nerve meets the retina, expanding the **blind spot**. "Papilloedema" is used to describe these changes in combination with raised intracranial pressure; when detected, intracranial mass should be considered (Lazaridou et al 2007). Other retinal hypertensive changes include cotton wool spots, arteriovenous clipping and shiny thickened artery walls- silver wiring.

93 – F

The visual phenomena are key, termed "**floaters**"- bright and dark spots and suggestive of **retinal detachment**. This occurs following a retinal tear, the vitreous humour separating the retina from the choroid. It is painless, can run in families, follow eye trauma and is more likely in middle-aged short-sighted people. Early retinal detachment may be treated using laser eye surgery or cryotherapy. Advanced detachment requires prompt open surgery. Once it develops in one eye, it is more likely contralaterally.

94 – H

Multiple sclerosis can present with **optic neuritis**, resulting in **eye pain** and **blurred vision**. This can progress to loss of colour vision or even monocular blindness. On fundoscopy, the optic disc appears pink and swollen if the nerve head is affected (papillitis, also caused by toxic amblyopia). Unlike papilloedema, papillitis may be unilateral, cause pain on eye movement, affect acuity early on, cause central scotomas (small areas outside blind spots of reduced vision) with intact venous pulsation. With retrobulbar neuritis, the optic nerve is affected behind the retina, such that fundoscopy is normal. There may also be a relative afferent papillary defect.

95 – E

The lateral visual field is focused upon the medial side of the retina and the medial field upon the lateral side. The nerves of the optic pathway from retina to V1 occipital cortex (via synapses at the lateral geniculate nucleus) maintain spatial relations according to their position on the retina (retinotopic). Optic nerve fibers originating from the medial retina decussate at the optic chiasm, thus each retina sends visual information to both occipital lobes and severing the optic pathway between the optic tract and V1 occipital cortex would cause hemianopia in both eyes affecting the contralateral visual hemifield. **Parietal lobe lesions** sever the superior fibers of the optic radiation (between geniculate nucleus and V1), causing **contralateral inferior homonymous quadrantanopias**. Temporal lesions affect inferior optic radiation fibres, causing contralateral superior homonymous quadrantanopia. Due to a protected blood supply, V1 CVAs tend to cause hemianopia with sparing of the macula (central) visual field.

Further Information (Q. 91 – 95)

Toxic amblyopia may manifest with sudden onset papillitis- swollen optic disc, reduced colour vision, impaired acuity, central scotoma. Causes include ingestion of quinine, tobacco, chloroquine and methyl alcohol (from contaminated alcohol). Amblyopia ex anopsia (AKA lazy eye) occurs when one eye is impaired from early childhood, often by cataracts or strabismus, leading the brain to ignore its input. Central retinal vein thrombosis results in haemorrhages across the whole retina, tortuous veins and disc swelling. Vitamin A, as 11-cis-retinal, is an essential component of the photosensitive pigment rhodopsin, found in rod photoreceptors and essential for sensitive low-detail (scotopic) night vision. Photoreceptor membranes break down on exposure to light; cone membranes are regenerated at night, rod membranes during the day, when each is less active. Vitamin A deficiency causes xerophthalmia, a group of eye conditions including night blindness, corneal ulceration and conjunctival xerosis. The WHO estimates 6-7 million new cases of xerophthalmia occur every year, 20% of which cause complete visual loss. Vitamin A deficiency is treated with retinol palmitate supplements orally or intramuscularly. Health education and mandatory food supplementation can eradicate Vitamin A deficiency, which also reduces MMR vaccine efficacy and increases the risk of vertical HIV transmission.

---

96 – D
Gabapentin is licensed for the treatment of diabetic neuropathy, as is duloxetine, a selective serotonin and noradrenaline reuptake inhibitor. Unlicensed treatments include amitriptyline and carbamazepine.

97 – H
The scenario suggests **giant cell arteritis,** needing immediate steroid treatment to prevent permanent visual loss, the **bisphosphonate alendronic acid** given to avoid steroid-induced osteoporosis. Amaurosis fugax is a sudden and normally temporary loss of vision due to vascular compromise of the retina. Causes include a thrombus from the left atrium in atrial fibrillation, fibrin or cholesterol crystals detached from carotid plaques and giant cell arteritis.

98 – C
Breakthrough pain occurs despite regular analgesic medication. Supplemental doses of morphine would act more slowly than **fentanyl,** an opioid that can be absorbed through the oral mucosa for rapid alleviation of breakthrough pain. The WHO proposes a 3 step pain management ladder, the 1st consisting of non-opioid analgesia. If this is not effective, the 2nd step is tried, consisting of mild opioids with or without non-opioids, while the 3rd consists of stronger opioid doses with or without non-opioids.

99 – A

Seconds-long bursts of facial pain suggest **trigeminal neuralgia.** Carbamazepine can reduce the intensity and frequency.

100 – E

The scenario suggests she is about to undergo **induction** of general anaesthesia. **Ketamine** blocks the NMDA glutamate receptor and is used for this purpose in **children** but less commonly in adults as it can cause psychosis and hypertension.

Further Information (Q. 96 – 100)

Melzack and Wall (1965) formulated the gate theory of pain, whereby afferent signals are modulated by desending signals at the spinal cord dorsal horn. Thus in painful conditions, whereby survival is threatened, endogenous serotonin or opioids diminish pain, enabling active (fight/ flight) or passive (playing dead) responses. When the danger has passed, the pain is no longer masked, increasing discomfort but preventing exacerbation of injuries. Codeine is a weak opiate used for mild to moderate pain and cough suppression. Morphine is a strong opiate used for severe pain. Tolfenamic acid is an NSAID for the treatment of acute migraine attack, an indication it shares with the 5HT-1 agonist sumatriptan.

4 Psychiatry EMQs

| 1 | Antipsychotic Drugs | PSYCHIATRY |

Options
A Aripiprazole
B Chlorpromazine
C Clozapine
D Flupentixol
E Fluphenazine
F Haloperidol
G Perphenazine
H Pimozide
I Risperidone
J Thioridazine

Select the most appropriate drug from the list above (each may be used once or more).

1. Mechanism relies on partial dopamine receptor agonism.

2. An atypical antipsychotic available in depot form.

3. The first neuroleptic developed, also can be used as an anti-emetic in palliative care.

4. Patients taking this drug require regular blood count monitoring.

5. Has the most marked sedating effect.

2	Self-harm	PSYCHIATRY

Options

A	Anorexia nervosa
B	Bipolar disorder
C	Borderline personality disorder
D	Depression
E	Dysthymia
F	Insomnia
G	Learning disability
H	Obsessive compulsive disorder
I	Post-traumatic stress disorder
J	Schizophrenia

Select the most appropriate diagnosis from the list above (each may be used once or more).

6. An 18-year-old female with history of childhood sexual abuse and volatile fluctuating mood expresses suicidal ideation.

7. A 42-year-old female repeatedly bites her upper lip, causing significant damage.

8. A 28-year-old male with recurring dreams cuts himself and displays passivity phenomena.

9. A 36-year-old female takes a paracetamol overdose after struggling with intrusive impulses, which she uses rituals to overcome.

10. An 18-year-old female with weight loss, early morning waking, low self-esteem, anhedonia and anergia takes an overdose.

| 3 | Drug abuse | PSYCHIATRY |

Options

A   Alcohol
B   Cannabis
C   Cocaine
D   Crack cocaine
E   Dexamphetamine
F   Ecstasy
G   Heroin
H   Methamphetamine
I   Poppers
J   Speedball

For each description below, select the single most likely drug of abuse from the list above (each may be used more than once):

11. Smoked stimulant that causes an intense high lasting 10-20 minutes, which can also be injected but not insufflated.

12. Prescription stimulant used at all-night raves, available as pills.

13. Orally active, injectable, insufflatable and inhalable stimulant made in home laboratories, containing substances from cold remedies.

14. Related compounds have been developed to treat nausea associated with chemotherapy.

15. Withdrawal causes visual hallucinations, formication, sweating, nausea, tachycardia, and convulsions.

| 4 | Drug treatment of schizophrenia | PSYCHIATRY |

Options
   A   Benperidol
   B   Clozapine
   C   Flumazenil
   D   Lorazepam
   E   Olanzapine
   F   Pimozide
   G   Procyclidine
   H   Pipotiazine
   I   Risperidone
   J   None of the above

For each scenario below select the single most appropriate antipsychotic drug. Each may be used more than once.

16.   A 35-year-old man with delusions of thought withdrawal and poor drug concordance requiring 2-weekly injections of a depot antipsychotic.

17.   An agitated 28-year-old man receiving treatment for schizophrenia who, for irrational reasons, is too frightened to leave the corner of his room.

18.   A feverish 70-year-old man who claims to see pigeons by his bed.

19.   A 24-year-old man whose delusions of thought insertion and paranoia have not abated after 4 months treatment, first with risperidone, then with quetiapine.

20.   A 31-year-old woman becomes more obese on first-line treatment for schizophrenia, which drug is likely to have caused this?

5	Physical symptoms	PSYCHIATRY

Options

A   Acute confusional state
B   Acute stress reaction
C   Alcohol withdrawal
D   Depression
E   Dissociative fugue
F   Paroxysmal anxiety
G   Post-traumatic stress disorder
H   Schizophrenia
I   Somatization disorder
J   None of the above

For each scenario below choose the single most appropriate diagnosis. Each may be used more than once.

21. A 44-year-old man distressed by sweating, tremor, visual and somatic hallucinations that developed 2 days after admission to hospital.

22. A 24-year-old man who remains in fixed poses after his limbs are passively moved.

23. A 37-year-old hypertensive obese woman with a history of depression, complaining of amenorrhoea, frontal balding, greasy skin, backache and weakness.

24. A 19-year-old man experiences anhedonia, autonomic hyperarousal, intrusive memories and recurrent nightmares. He says he needs alcohol to help him sleep.

25. A 48-year-old man suffers a sudden onset of crushing chest pain, sweating and dyspnoea while speaking on stage.

6	Treatment of depression	PSYCHIATRY

Options

A   Amitriptyline
B   Citalopram
C   Check concordance
D   Cognitive behavioural therapy
E   Electroconvulsive therapy
F   Increase dose
G   Paroxetine
H   Phenelzine
I   Reduce dose
J   Tryptophan

For each scenario, choose the single most appropriate treatment from the list above. Each may be used more than once.

26. A previously well 29-year-old woman with a 4-week onset of low mood, anergia, anhedonia, reduced self-esteem and no other symptoms.

27. A 31-year-old woman being treated for depression develops constipation and a dry mouth, what treatment is most likely to have caused this?

28. A 26-year-old man recovered from serious head injuries in a car crash before developing recurrent depression. Which option is likely to be contraindicated as augmentation of his paroxetine treatment?

29. A 16-year-old boy with low mood, anhedonia, anergia, early morning waking, low self-esteem and weight loss.

30. A 24-year-old woman with no response to 1 week's treatment with paroxetine.

| 7 | Duration of treatment and symptoms | PSYCHIATRY |

Options

A   Eight months
B   One month
C   One week
D   Six months
E   Six weeks
F   Ten weeks
G   Three months
H   Three weeks
I   Two weeks
J   Twelve weeks

For each treatment scenario, choose the most appropriate time period from the list above. Each may be used more than once.

31. A 29-year-old man with anergia, anhedonia, low mood, psychomotor agitation, and weight loss is started on imipramine, to which he responds. At least how long after remission of symptoms should treatment be continued for?

32. A 31 year-old woman has weight loss, anergia, early morning waking and low mood, how long do these symptoms generally have to be present for depression to be diagnosed?

33. A 22-year old man experiences thought echo auditory hallucinations. How long do these have to be present for schizophrenia to be diagnosed?

34. A 22-year-old man displays grandiosity, decreased need for sleep, recklessness and increased talkativeness that are disrupting his work life. How long do these usually have to be present for mania to be diagnosed?

35. A 19-year-old man with moderate depression is started on amitriptyline. After 3 weeks, he reports a partial response. How much longer should it be continued, assuming good concordance and tolerable side effects, before considering a change of medication?

8	Investigation	PSYCHIATRY

Questions

A   Creatine kinase, arterial blood gas, urea and electrolytes, urine myoglobin, clotting studies

B   Creatine kinase, urea and electrolytes, electrocardiogram,

C   Full blood count, liver function test, fasting blood glucose, lipid profile, electrocardiogram

D   Full blood count, bone marrow biopsy, urea and electrolytes

E   Full blood count, liver function test, serum HbA1c, urea and electrolytes

F   Full blood count, liver function test, urea and electrolytes

G   Full blood count, thyroid function test, clotting studies, arterial bood gas

H   Urea and electrolytes, urine myoglobulin, arterial blood gas

I   Urine and serum osmolality, serum drug level, urea and electrolytes

J   Thyroid function test, urea and electrolytes, serum drug level

For each scenario, choose the single most appropriate investigation(s) from the list above. Each may be used more than once.

36. A 37-year-old woman with bipolar disorder becomes drowsy, confused and polyuric.

37. A 32-year-old schizophrenic man prior to starting treatment with clozapine.

38. A 21-year-old man on long-term treatment with lithium for bipolar disorder, who has not had any blood tests for 6 months.

39. A 38-year-old man being treated for schizophrenia with haloperidol develops muscle rigidity, pyrexia, sweating and hypertension.

40. A 63-year-old depressed woman taking paroxetine develops diarrhoea, hypertension, mydriasis, pyrexia and tremor.

| 9 | Perpetual disturbance | PSYCHIATRY |

Options

A   Acute confusional state
B   Alcohol withdrawal
C   Bipolar disorder
D   Depressive stupor
E   Derealisation
F   Panic disorder
G   Partial seizure
H   Pseudohallucination
I   Schizophrenia
J   Severe depression

For each scenario, choose the single most likely diagnosis from the list above. Each may be used more than once.

41.   A 48-year-old man hears his own thoughts vocalised from his surroundings.

42.   A 33-year-old woman has several mystical episodes she cannot explain, each preceded by depersonalisation.

43.   A 72-year-old woman refuses to leave her house because of her offensive body odour, which she says remains despite repeated washing. You cannot smell anything.

44.   A 63-year-old agitated man receiving inpatient treatment, including sedatives, has tactile hallucinations.

45.   A 23-year-old agitated woman reports recent onset of hyperacusis and visual hyperaesthesia.

| 10 | Affective symptoms | PSYCHIATRY |

Options

A	Adjustment disorder
B	Atypical depression
C	Cushing's disease
D	Cyclothymia
E	Dementia
F	Hypothyroidism
G	Mild depression
H	Moderate depression
I	Schizophrenia
J	Severe depression

For each scenario, choose the single most likely diagnosis from the list above. Each may be used more than once.

46.   A 37-year-old woman with low mood worse in the morning, anergia, weight gain, constipation, impaired concentration and menorrhagia.

47.   A 69-year-old woman with low mood, who remains convinced that she has lost all her life savings, despite reassurances from her bank and family.

48.   A 23-year-old woman with anergia, weight loss, low mood, low self-esteem, suicidal ideation, anhedonia, psychomotor retardation, early morning waking, impaired concentration and a positive overnight dexamethasone suppression test.

49.   A 31-year-old man with low mood, reduced concentration, anergia and weight loss following a recent divorce.

50.   A 50-year-old man with increased appetite, anhedonia, low mood worse in the evenings, hypersomnia and fatigue.

| 11 | Perceptual Disorders | PSYCHIATRY |

Options

A   Complex auditory hallucination
B   Derealisation
C   Fantasy
D   Hypnogogic hallucination
E   Hypnopompic hallucination
F   Illusion
G   Macropsia
H   Pareidolia
I   Pseudohallucination
J   Visual hallucination

For each scenario, choose the single most likely phenomenon from the list above. Each may be used more than once.

51.   A 19-year-old man mistakes a tree silhouette for a person at night, realizing his error when he turns on his torch.

52.   A 49-year-old woman sees an image of her husband beckoning, 2 weeks after he died. She acknowledges there is nothing really there.

53.   A 32-year-old woman reads and understands a newspaper, but fails to notice several spelling mistakes.

54.   A 70-year-old woman hears an external voice giving a running commentary of her actions.

55.   A 5-year-old girl sees a fleeting image of a bear next to her bed on waking.

12	Social factors	PSYCHIATRY

Options
A   Afro-Caribbean racial group
B   Caring for 3 or more children aged less than 14
C   Chinese racial group
D   Education to secondary school level
E   Lost father at a young age
F   High socioeconomic class background
G   Lost mother at young age
H   Low socioeconomic class background
I   South Asian racial group
J   Victim of childhood sexual abuse

For each scenario, choose the single most likely associated social factor from the list above. Each may be used more than once.

56. A 30-year-old mentally ill man from a racial background in the UK-more likely to be admitted under the Mental Health Act.

57. A 22-year-old woman from a racial background in the UK with increased incidence of suicide amongst females.

58. A 23-year-old man with a history of conduct disorder and several convictions for violent offences which he explains were due to people picking on him because of his height.

59. A 21-year-old woman who is trying to further slim down despite being 40kg in weight, 155cm tall and amenorrhoeic.

60. A 22-year-old woman, who tends to form intense but unstable and chaotic personal relationships, with a tendency to make threats of self-harm.

13	Personality disorders	PSYCHIATRY

Options

A   Anankastic
B   Antisocial
C   Anxious
D   Borderline
E   Dependent
F   Histrionic
G   Impulsive
H   Narcissistic
I   Paranoid
J   Schizoid

For each scenario, choose the single most likely personality disorder from the list above. Each may be used more than once.

61. A 29-year-old man working in an insurance claims department who lives alone. He writes prodigiously but is not concerned about being recognised in his lifetime and has little need of company.

62. A 38-year-old man frequently alludes to unsuccessful job interviews, believing that they are the reason he lacks confidence and some of his friends no longer talk to him.

63. A 32-year-old actor given to volatile moods who is less happy when people in his company are not talking about him. He lends himself to expansive gestures of affection or sometimes enmity when he sees colleagues.

64. A 26-year-old woman who intricately schedules her day, most of which is spent working as an astrophysicist, leaving her little time to pursue other interests. Decisions in her work and social life are excessively mulled over.

65. A 35-year-old man working as an auditor who has pursued five employment tribunals, one of which was successful. His home life has been disrupted several times in the past by him accusing his wife of infidelity.

14	Delusions	PSYCHIATRY

Options
A   Delusional disorder
B   Delusional memory
C   Delusional mood
D   Delusional perception
E   Delusion of control
F   Delusion of passivity
G   Delusion of thought broadcast
H   Delusion of thought insertion
I   Delusion of thought withdrawal
J   Secondary delusion

For each scenario, choose the single most likely type of delusion from the list above. Each may be used more than once.

66. A 69-year-old man with a reduced need for sleep explains volubly how he has the power to control the weather.

67. A 32-year-old woman deduces that an attack of malaria she had as a child was the first of many assassination attempts.

68. 39-year-old man believes his memories are being intercepted by the military dictatorship of Myanmar.

69. A 22-year-old man blames himself personally for starting a fatal house fire reported in Bolton, despite reassurances that he has never been there.

70. A 34-year-old woman reports an abnormal feeling, as if something was about to happen.

15	Organic psychiatry	PSYCHIATRY

Options

A   44 CAG repeats on chromosome 4

B   Beta amyloid plaque deposition, neurofibrillary tangles and atrophy at the hippocampus

C   Mother had rubella during gestation

D   MRI scan shows enlarged lateral ventricles, subtle atrophy at medial temporal, lateral temporal and prefrontal lobes. Increased dopamine release in mesolimbic system

E   MRI shows reduction in volume of orbitofrontal cortex

F   Positive 48-hour dexamathesone suppression test.

G   Positive overnight dexamethasone suppression test, mildly elevated TSH, CSF 5-hydroxyindoleacetic acid (5-HIAA) low

H   Positive overnight dexamethasone suppression test, mildly elevated TSH, MRI scan shows evidence of a clinically silent CVA

I   T2 MRI shows periventricular areas of oedema and demyelination

J   T2 MRI shows reduced volume of mamillary bodies.

For each scenario, choose the single most likely physiological findings from the list above. Each may be used more than once.

71.   A 27-year-old depressed woman who is brought to hospital after surviving an attempt to hang herself.

72.   A 21year-old man who spoke his first word aged 6, shows little interest in others and gets upset if his day is slightly disrupted.

73.   A 32-year-old man makes a series of impulsive financial and relationship misjudgements, following brain damage. His intelligence is intact.

74.   A 34-year-old man claims a Colombian drugs cartel is plotting to kill him. He knows this because he saw a poster for a salsa event.

75.   A 35-year-old man with a long-term alcohol problem and anterograde amnesia.

| 16 | Eponymous syndromes | PSYCHIATRY |

Options

A   Alice in Wonderland syndrome
B   Asperger's syndrome
C   Capgras syndrome
D   Cotard's syndrome
E   De Clerambault's syndrome
F   Fregoli's syndrome
G   Munchausen's syndrome
H   Tourette's syndrome
I   Wernicke-Korsakoff's syndrome
J   None of the above

For each scenario, choose the single most likely eponymous syndrome from the list above. Each may be used more than once.

76. A 31-year-old man is convinced he has met his mother in the street. She is adamant that they are strangers.

77. A 44-year-old man reacts with denial followed by fresh sadness on hearing about his mother's death 2 weeks ago. However, family members say that he went to her funeral.

78. A 73-year-old woman with anhedonia, early morning waking and weight loss believes that she is already dead.

79. A 6-year-old boy with a learning disability cannot speak any words (despite having good hearing), lacks sociability and has stereotyped interests.

80. A 36-year-old man says that he is following a famous rapper around the country because she is in love with him. She has tried to obtain a restraining order.

17	Learning disability	PSYCHIATRY

Options
A   Cerebral palsy
B   Down syndrome
C   Fetal alcohol syndrome
D   Fragile X syndrome
E   Neurofibromatosis
F   Phenylketonuria
G   Prader-Willi syndrome
H   Rett's syndrome
I   Rubella embryopathy
J   Tuberous sclerosis

For the learning disability scenarios below, pick the most appropriate diagnosis from the choices above. Each may be used more than once.

81.   A 4-year-old boy with delayed uptake of language and a fear of social contact, who likes to arrange toy cars in a particular alignment and becomes upset if this is disrupted. His testicles have a volume of 4ml and he has large ears.

82.   A 2-year-old growth-retarded girl with small eyes, facial deformities and language difficulties who is being evaluated for special needs. Neither of her parents has learning disabilities.

83.   A 3-month-old infant born with several defects including microcephaly, cataracts and a ventricular septal defect.

84.   An 8-year-old boy in a mainstream primary school with a flat occiput and single palmar crease.

85.   A 3-year-old girl with previously normal development who loses her ability to speak and her hand co-ordination skills.

18	Overdose and substance abuse	PSYCHIATRY

Options
A   Activated charcoal
B   Alcohol
C   Apomorphine
D   Buprenorphine
E   Disulfiram
F   Flumazenil
G   Methadone
H   N-acetyl cysteine
I   Naloxone
J   Naltrexone

For the poisoning and substance abuse scenarios below, choose the most appropriate treatment from the list above. Each may be used more than once.

86. A 15-year-old girl is admitted in a state of reduced consciousness after ingesting antifreeze several hours ago.

87. A 28-year-old male heroin addict is admitted with reduced consciousness and pinpoint pupils. Though naloxone is initially helpful, he deteriorates within minutes.

88. A 63-year-old male with vomiting, abdominal pain and bruising, admitted with paracetamol overdose several hours ago.

89. A 45-year-old female recovering problem drinker who would benefit from first-line treatment to reduce the likelihood of relapse.

90. A 31-year-old female recovering heroin addict who is no longer dependent and would benefit from treatment to reduce the likelihood of relapse.

| 19 | Prevalence and predisposition | PSYCHIATRY |

Options

A	~ 0.01%
B	~ 0.05%
C	~ 0.1%
D	~ 1%
E	~ 3%
F	10-20%
G	20-30%
H	30-40%
I	40-50%
J	50-60%

For the scenarios below, pick the most accurate percentage from above. Each may be used more than once.

91. What is the prevalence of borderline personality disorder amongst women in the UK?

92. What is the yearly risk of suicide for a UK prison inmate?

93. What is the lifetime prevalence of schizophrenia in Jamaica?

94. What is the lifetime prevalence of a female in the UK developing bipolar affective disorder?

95. What proportion of UK men drink more than the maximum safe daily limit of alcohol at least once in a week?

20	Mental Health Act	PSYCHIATRY

Options

    A   Section 2
    B   Section 3
    C   Section 4
    D   Section 5(4)
    E   Section 35
    F   Section 37
    G   Section 48
    H   Section 58
    I   Section 59
    J   Section 136

For the scenarios below, pick the most appropriate section from the list above.

96. The police bring a vulnerable 22-year-old woman, found wandering the streets claiming to be an angel, to a psychiatric unit.

97. A nurse wishes to detain an agitated 26-year-old man, in hospital with a rib fracture, for psychiatric assessment. A doctor is not available.

98. Two psychiatric registrars and a social worker agree on a compulsory 6 month admission of a psychotic 33-year-old man.

99. A psychiatric team seek special consent for a cingulotomy operation on a man with intractable, debilitating obsessive compulsive disorder.

100. A judge and 2 psychiatrists agree that a mentally ill man accused of assault requires compulsory admission to a psychiatric hospital, as opposed to gaol, for a minimum of 6 months.

5 Psychiatry EMQs Answers & Explanations

Quick Answers

1	A	2	I	3	B	4	C	5	B
6	C	7	G	8	J	9	H	10	D
11	D	12	E	13	H	14	B	15	A
16	I	17	D	18	J	19	B	20	E
21	C	22	H	23	J	24	G	25	J
26	D	27	A	28	E	29	B	30	C
31	D	32	I	33	B	34	C	35	H
36	I	37	C	38	J	39	A	40	A
41	I	42	G	43	J	44	B	45	C
46	F	47	J	48	J	49	G	50	B
51	F	52	I	53	F	54	A	55	E
56	A	57	I	58	J	59	F	60	J
61	J	62	C	63	F	64	A	65	I
66	J	67	B	68	I	69	J	70	C
71	G	72	C	73	E	74	D	75	J
76	F	77	I	78	D	79	J	80	E
81	D	82	C	83	I	84	B	85	H
86	B	87	I	88	H	89	E	90	J
91	E	92	C	93	D	94	D	95	H
96	J	97	D	98	B	99	I	100	F

Explanations

1 – A

Aripiprazole is a licensed atypical antipsychotic (AKA neuroleptic) which is said to alleviate both positive and negative symptoms of schizophrenia, acting as a partial dopamine receptor agonist and antagonist.

2 – I

Risperidone is the first atypical to be available in depot form. Depot injections of antipsychotics are administered intramuscularly and can also be given monthly. They are more likely to be used in patients with concordance problems but may negate patient autonomy.

3 – B

Chlorpromazine was the first antipsychotic licensed, in 1954. Chlorpromazine, flupentixol, fluphenazine, haloperidol, perphenazine, pimozide and thioridazine are all typical antipsychotic drugs, meaning their method of action relies on blocking the D2 dopamine receptor. Blocking the D2 receptor at the chemoreceptor trigger zone reduces nausea.

4 – C

Clozapine is an antipsychotic reserved for treatment-resistant cases because of its side-effects, including ~0.8% risk of agranulocytosis, ~3% risk of neutropenia, fatal myocarditis, cardiomyopathy, diabetes mellitus and GI pseudo-obstruction. Blood dyscrasias are more likely in the elderly and those with benign essential neutropenia (commoner in those of West African origin). Before prescribing, a full medical history, physical examination and FBC are required, with possible further investigations and FBC monitoring and surveillance by the Clozaril patient monitoring service (UK).

5 – B

Chlorpromazine is the most sedating drug listed, with rapid effects, which can be useful in treating violent patients.

Further Information (Q. 1 – 5)

Perphenazine's other indications include use as an anti-emetic. ECG's are recommended before prescribing pimozide, due to the risk of arrhythmias. Thioridazine also requires ECG and is only prescribed under specialist supervision.

6 – C

Childhood abuse may predispose to borderline personality disorder and depression so the key phrase is **fluctuating mood- borderline personality** causes volatile moods, insecurity, problems with trust and abandonment fears that make forming stable close relationships difficult. Bipolar disorder causes mood variation with longer, more pronounced peaks and troughs than implied in the scenario.

7 – G

People with trouble expressing emotional pain may self-harm and this includes those with **learning disabilities**. Such a disfigurement is more likely in a person with a weaker understanding of self-image.

8 – J

The dreams are irrelevant, **passivity phenomena** (AKA delusions of passivity aka delusions of control) are the belief that an external force is controlling your body, one of Schneider's first rank symptoms of **schizophrenia**. The others are delusions of thought possession (insertion/broadcast/ withdrawal), auditory hallucinations in 3rd person thought echo and delusional perception (a real perception acquires a deluded interpretation e.g. seeing a butterfly means the police are following you).

9 – H

The intrusive thoughts are obsessions, which she would rather avoid, for example of violence or contamination. Compulsive rituals such as handwashing or counting, which may or may not be related to the obsession, are used to overcome these unpleasant thoughts. Rituals may temporarily alleviate discomfort, but in the long-term perpetuate the obsessions by reinforcing the anxious reaction they generate. The person would know these acts are illogical, possibly trying to conceal them. Up to 10% of obsessive compulsive people attempt suicide at some point.

10 – D

Anhedonia is the loss of pleasure in previously enjoyed activities, **anergia** is extreme lethargy. These are 2 of the 3 core ICD-10 features of **depression**, (the other being sustained low mood) which along with weight loss, **early-morning waking** (particularly suggestive of depression) and low self-esteem (non-core features) sustained for 2 weeks or more meet the criteria for depression. Unspecified weight loss and low self-esteem without a false body image or endocrine disturbance **do not** constitute anorexia nervosa.

Further Information (Q. 6 – 10)

Insomnia is classed by ICD-10 as a behavioural disorder, which means that organic, drug-induced, psychotic, affective and anxiety-related diagnoses are considered beforehand to explain a lack of sleep. Dysthymia is a longer-lasting form of low mood which does not fit the criteria of depression.

---

11 – D

Crack cocaine produces a short-lived high followed by depression, paranoia, vomiting and muscle cramps. It is an extremely addictive class A drug, which can be injected after dissolving it in acid, but cannot be insufflated (snorted). Cocaine can be smoked or injected, but is primarily insufflated. Methamphetamine and heroin can be eaten, smoked, insufflated or injected but produce longer highs.

12 – E

The key word is "**prescription**". **Dexamphetamine** is sometimes prescribed for attention deficit hyperactivity disorder, in patients not responding to methylphenidate. Dexamphetamine was used by northern soul dancers (hence the band name "Dexys Midnight Runners"); ecstasy is a dance drug but is not prescribed.

13 – H

The class A drug **Methamphetamine** is a modified form of speed (amphetamine). Home laboratories are dangerous due to the flammable and toxic phosphine fumes produced, causing burns and respiratory problems. Cold and allergy remedies contain minute amounts of ephedrine or pseudoephedrine, which cause vasoconstriction to relieve nasal congestion.

14 – B

Nabilone is a cannabinoid appetite stimulant developed for this purpose. Recreational cannabis use can also have this effect.

15 – A

The key terms are **visual hallucinations** and particularly **convulsions**, which suggest alcohol rather than heroin, methamphetamine or cocaine withdrawal. **Alcohol** withdrawal can lead to delirium tremens, a reduced state of consciousness characterised by tachycardia, sweating, tremors, nausea, convulsions, tactile and visual hallucinations. It is managed with a reducing dose regimen of the benzodiazepine chlordiazepoxide;without treatment, the mortality rate is up to 10%. Therefore, when a history hints at alcohol dependency, it is very important to prescribe a detox regimen for the admitted patient, even on the PRN (as required) side of the drug chart.

Further Information (Q. 11 – 15)

Speedball is an injected mixture of heroin and cocaine. Poppers is a name for amyl nitrite, a legal drug (toxic when swallowed), which on inhalation causes light-headedness, anal sphincter relaxation and headaches. Medically it is used to treat cyanide poisoning and angina. Heroin use causes constipation, euphoria, analgesia, respiratory depression, constricted pupils and reduced consciousness. Heroin withdrawal has the opposite effects, leading to diarrhoea, intense craving, pain, abdominal cramps, sweating, running nose and eyes, unstable temperature control, dilated pupils, with insomnia and restlessness, beginning ~6 hours after the last dose and peaking at ~36-48 hours. Unlike alcohol withdrawal, opiate withdrawal tends not to cause visual or tactile hallucinations and mortality is relatively rare. Symptoms of opiate withdrawal can be ameliorated by a reducing dose of methadone, with urine tests for other drug use. Dirty needles cause infectious endocarditis and cerebral abscesses. Sharing injecting paraphernalia transmits HIV, Hepatitis B, C and D; which was reduced by the introduction of needle exchanges to UK pharmacies.

16 – I

The answer is **risperidone** as it is the only atypical neuroleptic currently available by depot. NICE (2002) recommends all newly-diagnosed people with schizophrenia are treated with atypical neuroleptics as they cause fewer extra-pyramidal side-effects. .

17 – D

For psychotic behaviour like this, the **sedative** effect of IV or oral **lorazepam** (a benzodiazepine) is useful. More dangerous agitation can indicate haloperidol and lorazepam by intramuscular injection.

18 – J
Antipsychotics are to be used with caution in the **elderly**. His fever and visual hallucination suggest an organic cause, making acute **confusional state** more likely than schizophrenia; the cause of his **fever** should be treated.

19 – B
Clozapine should only be prescribed when schizophrenia is **inadequately controlled despite the sequential use of 2 or more antipsychotics**, one of which should be an atypical, each for at least 6-8 weeks (NICE 2002).

20 – E
Olanzapine and clozapine are more strongly associated with weight gain than risperidone (Wirshing et al 1999). First-line treatment of newly-diagnosed schizophrenia should be atypical antipsychotics, such as amisulpride, aripipirazole, olanzapine, quetiapine, **risperidone**, sertindole and zotepine (NICE 2002), which have fewer extra-pyramidal side-effects than typical antipsychotics. Clozapine also can cause weight gain, but although atypical is not first-line due to its hazardous side-effects. Olanzepine and risperidone cause anticholinergic effects like worsening angle closure glaucoma.

Further Information (Q. 16 – 20)
Prescribing more than one antipsychotic simultaneously is not recommended, apart from during transition between regimens. Although NICE (2002) recommends atypical antipsychotics for newly-diagnosed schizophrenic patients, it is not recommended to change medication for those adequately treated by typical antipsychotics. Benperidol is a typical neuroleptic sometimes used to curb predatory sexual behaviour. Flumazenil is a benzodiazepine antagonist used in treatment of overdose. Procyclidine is an anticholinergic used to ameliorate drug-induced Parkinsonian symptoms, apart from tardive dyskinesia. Pipotiazine is a phenothiazine typical neuroleptic available by depot.

---

21 – C
Although **visual and somatic hallucinations** are possible in schizophrenia, they are characteristic of **alcohol withdrawal**, typically seeing small objects like spiders in the peripheral vision and feeling insects crawling

under the skin (formication). The benzodiazepine chlordiazepoxide is used to prevent delirium tremens.

22 – H

This is **waxy flexibility** (cerea flexibilitas). The limbs offer resistance then remain moulded in a posture, a feature characteristic of catatonic **schizophrenia**.

23 – J

These are all features of **Cushing's disease**, due to an excess of corticosteroids, either from drugs or hormone-secreting tumours.

24 – G

Following an ordeal like rape or war, **post-traumatic stress disorder** may cause **flashbacks**, emotional blunting and avoidance of activities that may remind the person of their experience. **Autonomic hyperarousal** is a persisting crisis response, with features like exaggerated startle response and insomnia. To cope with these symptoms, people may abuse drugs. **Anhedonia** is the loss of pleasure in previously enjoyed activities and is also a core feature of depression. Treatments for post-traumatic stress disorder include antidepressants, talking therapies and eye-movement desensitization and reprocessing (EMDR).

25 – J

Though a **sudden-onset** of **crushing chest pain**, **sweating** and **dyspnoea** can be features of paroxysmal anxiety, **myocardial infarction** should be first considered.

Further Information (Q. 21 – 25)

According to the ICD-10 diagnostic hierarchy, organic conditions then drug-induced symptoms must be considered before psychiatric illnesses. Somatization disorder is the persistence of multiple medically unexplainable symptoms, often in many body systems, with demands for multiple investigations. ICD-10 stipulates it must have at least a 2 year history, have no adequate physical explanation, cause a functional impairment and be accompanied by the refusal to accept reassurances.

Dissociative fugue is amnesia for an unpleasant memory combined with an increased amount of purposeful travel and maintenance of normal social interaction.

Acute confusional state is caused by organic illness or drugs and characterised by diminished consciousness with impaired cognition and possible hallucinations, mood changes and physical signs like fever.

Acute stress reaction is an abnormal and disproportionate emotional response to stressful events, which may feature generalised anxiety and panic attacks (paroxysmal anxiety).

---

26 – D
This constitutes **4 features**, classed as **mild depression**, for which antidepressant side-effects are likely to outweigh benefits. Treatments include **cognitive behavioural therapy**, exercise programmes, counselling and problem-solving therapy.

27 – A
Amitriptyline is the most likely, as a tricyclic antidepressant, to have caused the anti-cholinergic side-effects mentioned. At the heart, these can include tachycardia, arrhythmias, and hypotension. Tricyclics can cause pupillary dilatation with impaired accommodation and worsening closed-angle glaucoma. There may also be urinary retention and confusion, while alpha adrenoreceptor blocking effects include postural hypotension, erectile dysfunction and drowsiness.

28 – E
The implied history of intracranial haemorrhage precludes treatment with **electroconvulsive therapy**. (NICE 2007).

29 – B
SSRIs are recommended for initial treatment of moderate to severe depression (this is moderate). They are recommended over tricyclics due to the smaller risk of side-effects halting treatment (NICE 2007). **Citalopram** is the answer because paroxetine is not recommended for under-18's (CSM 2003), due to increased risk of self-harming behaviour. Other side-effects of SSRI's include restlessness, agitation, serotonin syndrome, insomnia, restlessness, tremor, ejaculatory delay.

30 – C
Non-concordance is a major reason for treatment failure, normally checked after **1 week** of paroxetine treatment. It is important to empha-

sise its importance, since up to 6 weeks may pass before effects occur. If treatment fails despite good concordance, in the absence of major side-effects, doses may be increased.

Further Information (Q. 26 – 30)

Antidepressant Drug Class	Examples
Tricyclic antidepressants	Amitriptyline, clomipramine, dothiepin, imipramine.
Specific serotonin reuptake inhibitors	Citalopram, fluoxetine, paroxetine, sertraline.
Serotonin-noradrenaline reuptake inhibitor	Venlafaxine
Selective noradrenaline reuptake inhibitor	Reboxetine.
Reversible monoamine oxidase inhibitors	Moclobemide
Irreversible monoamine oxidase inhibitors	Phenelzine, isocarboxazid
Other	Mianserin, mirtazepine (α2 adrenoreceptor blocker)
Augmentation of antidepressants	Lithium, electroconvulsive therapy, tryptophan, flupentixol

Tricyclic antidepressants, specific serotonin reuptake inhibitors, and moclobemide (a reversible monoamine oxidase inhibitor) all have the same efficacy (with full concordance) of 60%-70%. Antidepressants are recommended for moderate to severe depression (NICE 2007), with SSRI's recommended as first-line.

Treatment duration is at least 6 months after remission of symptoms, reducing dose over ~4 weeks at termination. With persistent treatment-resistant depression, 2 drugs may be tried simultaneously if the patient is willing to tolerate the increased risk of side-effects.

Monoamine oxidase inhibitors like phenelzine can cause the "**cheese reaction**", whereby tyramine, a monoamine found in cheese and chocolate is not metabolised. At neurones it displaces monoamines, leading to a rapid and potentially fatal rise in blood pressure. To avoid this, people taking monoamine oxidase inhibitors (even irreversible forms) are warned not to eat large amounts of mature cheese, yeast extracts or fermented soy bean extracts and should not be given sympathomimetic drugs (BNF 2008).

Tryptophan is an essential amino acid, required to produce serotonin. It is prescribed by specialists as an adjunct in severe treatment-resistant depression; tryptophan- depleted diets have been shown to worsen depression in patients receiving treatment (Delgado et al 1990).

31 – D
Six months is the minimum antidepressant treatment recommended for a patient of this age (NICE 2007).

32 – I
According to ICD-10 symptoms should be present for **2 weeks** to diagnose **depression**, though it can be diagnosed sooner with more severe or of rapid onset.

33 – B
According to ICD-10, schizophrenic symptoms lasting less than **1 month** are termed "acute schizophrenic-like psychotic disorder", with the term "**schizophrenia**" only used for episodes longer than this. With DSM-IV, the minimum duration is 6 months, before which the symptoms are termed "schizophreniform".

34 – C
According to ICD-10, symptoms should be present a minimum of **1 week** before a **manic** episode is diagnosed, though again if they are unusually severe a shorter time period is allowed.

35 – H
With partial response, six weeks are given before antidepressant therapy is changed, meaning **3 more weeks** are required (NICE 2007).

Further Information (Q. 31 – 35)
Stopping treatment abruptly or too early can produce a rebound depression more severe than the original complaint and this should be strongly advised against. SSRI's may cause anxiety symptoms in the first 2 weeks of treatment and take up to 6 weeks to exert their full effects. If no response is seen after 1 week, concordance should be checked. If this is good, the dose may be increased or a new drug tried.

36 – I

Lithium is used in the prophylaxis of bipolar depression and it can cause **diabetes insipidus**, the lack of ADH action at the kidney. **Increased serum osmolality** and **reduced urine osmolality** would be expected, with **elevated serum lithium** levels and **hyponatremia** predisposing to lithium toxicity. Other side-effects include tremor, mental slowing, weight gain and hypothyroidism.

37 – C

Due to its side effects, a full medical history, blood pressure, weight, examination, **FBC**, LFT, lipid profile, fasting blood glucose and ECG are recommended before starting **clozapine**. If cardiac abnormalities are found, specialist advice is sought before starting treatment.

38 – J

Serum lithium measurements are required every 3-6 months, **TFTs** every 6-12 months alongside regular **renal function** tests when on long-term treatment.

39 – A

This suggests **neuroleptic malignant syndrome**, which though rare, can be fatal, for example through respiratory failure, myoglobinuric renal failure, acute heart failure and hyperthermia leading to disseminated intravascular coagulation. Like extrapyramidal side-effects, it is more likely with **typical antipsychotics** such as haloperidol, which work by blocking dopamine D_2 receptors, than atypical antipsychotics. Elevated **Creatine kinase** indicates muscle damage which can lead to rhabdomyolysis and renal failure, which would be detected by the **U & E** and **urine myoglobin** tests; **ABG** would pick up metabolic acidosis. Chest x ray, lumbar puncture, sputum and blood cultures may be indicated if sepsis is suspected.

40 – A

These features suggest the rare but potentially fatal serotonin syndrome, which can be caused by SSRI's. Like neuroleptic malignant syndrome, there may be rhabdomyolysis, acute renal failure, disseminated intravascular coagulation, metabolic acidosis which **U&E, urine myoglobin, creatine kinase, clotting studies**, and **ABG** can detect. However, SSRI's have generally fewer anti-muscarinic, sedating and cardiotoxic effects than tricyclic antidepressants, and for this reason are recommended as first-line treatment (NICE 2007).

Further Information (Q. 36 – 40)

Neuroleptic malignant syndrome: a life-threatening condition featuring hyperthermia, tachycardia, sweating, convulsions, reduced consciousness, muscle rigidity and hypertension which develop within 4-10 days of starting typical antipsychotics. If it occurs, treatment is stopped, dantrolene given as a muscle relaxant and bromocriptine may be used to counter antipsychotic dopamine receptor blockage. The patient should be kept cool, with monitoring of blood pressure, pulse rate, temperature, U&E, CK, urine myoglobin, clotting.

Tardive dyskinesia: involuntary and purposeless movements like lip-smacking, jaw movements and tongue protrusion, seen with long-term antipsychotic treatment and exacerbated by anticholinergic drugs. Benzodiazepines may help, or careful transfer to atypical antipsychotics, but tardive dyskinesia can be a chronic debilitating problem, remaining after treatment is withdrawn.

Acute dystonia: involuntary sustained contractions, usually within 3 days of starting antipsychotic treatment. This can be treated with anticholinergics, reducing the dose or switching to an atypical. It can also be caused by SSRI's, anticonvulsants, dopamine agonists and metoclopramide.

Akathisia: a feeling of restlessness and unease which tends to occur within 1 to 10 weeks of starting antipsychotics. It may be treated with propranolol, a short course of diazepam or reducing the dose if possible.

---

41 – I

This is a **thought echo**, a first-rank symptom of **schizophrenia**.

42 – G

Mystical experiences can be caused by **temporal lobe epilepsy**; organic and drug-induced states should be considered before diagnosing psychotic illness. Treating this as schizophrenia could worsen symptoms as many antipsychotics reduce seizure threshold. **Depersonalisation** occurs as an aura prior to the seizure, causing a feeling of self-detachment, like mind and body becoming separate.

43 – J

This is a **mood-congruent olfactory hallucination**, encountered with **severe depression**.

44 – B

The **tactile hallucination** is **formication**, feeling ants crawling under the skin, caused by alcohol and cocaine withdrawal. This can occur in spite of chlordiazepoxide treatment, perhaps if the dose is insufficient, or treatment has just started.

45 – C

Increased sensitivity to sound and colour are features of manic phase **bipolar disorder**.

Further Information (Q. 41 – 45)

Psychosis is defined as a gross impairment of reality testing, in the absence of organic or drug-related causes. Psychotic people have trouble distinguishing their perceptual disturbances (e.g. hallucinations and delusions) from genuine external stimuli. Somatic hallucinations can be tactile, kinaesthetic (involving position sense, the feeling of limbs being moved), or visceral (e.g. feeling rats moving in the stomach) and are associated with increased risk of self-harm. Olfactory (smell) hallucinations often are strongly mood-related. Gustatory (taste) hallucinations are very rare, and non-psychiatric causes are more likely, such as benzodiazepines causing a lingering metallic taste. Acute confusional state involves reduced cognitive ability and decreased consciousness level, often featuring visual hallucinations or illusions. Temporal lobe epilepsy can mimic the auditory hallucinations of schizophrenia. Hallucinations may also be caused by sensory deprivation. Derealisation makes the patient's surroundings feel dreamlike and can occur with sleep deprivation. Depressive stupor occurs with severe depression and features a conscious but unresponsive state, with loss of speech and minimal movement.

46 – F

Although more obvious features like goitre, hair thinning, slow-relaxing reflexes, peripheral oedema and skin changes are not mentioned, all the mentioned features can be caused by **hypothyroidism**, an organic condition to be considered before depression. TFT would be performed to confirm or exclude this.

47 – J
She has a **delusion of poverty**, a **mood-congruent psychosis** encountered in **severe depression**.

48 – J
The overnight dexamethasone suppression test is a **screening investigation** for Cushing's disease, it has a ~12.5% false positive rate and ~50% of severely depressed patients test false positive. She has **9 features of depression** and no features specific to Cushing's (though it can cause depression). Features suggesting Cushing's as opposed to depression include skin darkening (if ACTH is increased), bitemporal hemianopia (pituitary tumour compressing the optic chiasm), acne, moon face, buffalo hump, osteoporosis, impaired wound healing, increased infection risk, skin thinning, purpura and muscle wasting. The 48-hour dexamethasone suppression test is more specific and could be performed to finalise the diagnosis, with depression considered more likely so far.

49 – G
A history of divorce does not exclude **mild depression** in favour of adjustment disorder when he has the diagnostic features.

50 – B
The features of **overeating, mood worse in the evening** and **hypersomnia** suggest **atypical depression**.

Further Information (Q. 46 – 50)
When psychotic depression and schizophrenia both seem possible, the presence of Schneider first rank symptoms of schizophrenia, the order in which symptoms presented and the affective quality of psychiatric features should be considered. In schizoaffective disorder, affective and psychotic features alternate at equal intensity. Biological phenomena found in severe depression include decreased plasma tryptophan, decreased plasma 5-hydroxytryptamine (serotonin), reduced noradrenaline-mediated release of growth hormone, subclinical hypothyroidism. Adjustment disorder occurs when a life change causes more distress than would normally be expected; occurring within 1 month of the change, while not meeting criteria for depression or anxiety. Precipitating events can include loss of a job, divorce but not bereavement; treatment focuses on talking therapies.

51 – F
Illusions are misperceptions of external stimuli and are more likely when sensory input is reduced, e.g. in the dark.

52 – I
Pseudohallucinations are not felt as real, though the stimulus may seem vivid, the patient recognises they are false. They are common following bereavement.

53 – F
This is an example of a **completion illusion**, in which **aspects of the external environment are subconsciously filled in**. With this phenomenon, only a small proportion of incident light hits the colour-sensitive part of the retina (fovea) and yet we perceive colour in our peripheral vision, facilitated by the V4 visual cortex region, damage to which produces achromotopsia. With this condition, the surroundings are only perceived in shades of grey; people thus afflicted are more vulnerable to depression and loss of appetite.

54 – A
This is **third person auditory hallucination**, a suggestive feature of **schizophrenia**.

55 – E
Hypnopompic hallucinations appear briefly on waking, **hypnogogic hallucinations** appear briefly on the approach of sleep. They are not abnormal.

Further Information (Q. 51 – 55)
Pareidolia is a perceptual phenomenon in which existing external sensory cues are combined with imaginative input. Elementary auditory hallucinations are simpler than voices, for example rattling or machinery whir and are more associated with organic disease than psychiatric. Someone complaining of voices from inside their head is not strictly suffering hallucinations, because hallucinations are perceived as external and real; voices from inside the head are classed pseudohallucinations. According to psychoanalytic theory, distressing unconscious fantasies can lead to psychological symptoms. Macropsia is a perceptual disturbance causing objects to appear bigger than they are; this can result from organic retinal disease, complex partial epilepsy and migraines.

56 – A

In the UK, people from the **Afro-Caribbean racial group** are more likely to be compulsorily detained under the 1983 Mental Health Act, be described as violent, detained on secure units, receive physical treatments and be attended by junior rather than consultant staff (Hillier 1997, NIMH 2003). Elevated rates of compulsory admission, physical treatment and suicide have also been found amongst Irish-born people in the UK (NIMH 2003).

57 – I

South Asian (as well as Irish) women in Britain have been found to have a higher rate of suicide than women from other backgrounds (NIMH 2003). Overall, women have a lower age-standardised suicide rate than men, at 17.3 and 5.3 per 100 000 respectively in 2006 (Office for National Statistics).

58 – J

This is a description of **antisocial personality disorder**, which features a disregard for the feelings of others and the law, an inability to maintain relationships and a lack of remorse. Prevalence is ~1% (mainly men), reaching 15-25% in prison (Hare 1991).

Conduct disorder as a child is said to precede antisocial personality disorder in all cases, though only ~50% of children with conduct disorder develop antisocial disorder. Such people are said to have a tendency to blame other people and society for their actions.

However, it is also acknowledged that antisocial personality disorder is **predisposed by social disadvantages** such as parental substance abuse, being a victim of **child physical or sexual abuse** and being brought up in Care. Prevalence is ~1% (mainly men), reaching 15-25% in prison (Hare 1991).

59 – F

These constitute the **3 ICD-10 features** required for a diagnosis of **anorexia nervosa**, which is more prevalent amongst white females from higher socio-economic classes in Western countries. However, nearly all diseases, including schizophrenia and depression are more common with social deprivation, comparing socioeconomic class V to I.

60 – J

This is a description of **borderline personality disorder**, which is predisposed to by childhood adversity such as physical abuse, sexual abuse and neglect. Parents of such people are more likely to have borderline personality, antisocial personality, alcoholism and affective disorders. Childhood sexual abuse may also predispose to subsequent substance abuse, depression, anxiety and post-traumatic stress disorder.

Further Information (Q. 56 – 60)

The "social drift" hypothesis proposes that schizophrenia clusters in lower social classes because it causes functional impairment before the onset of psychosis, while the "environmental breeder" hypothesis conversely proposes that social adversity in childhood increases the risk. Fearon et al (2006) found a 6.8 risk ratio for Afro-Caribbean people and 5.6 for Black African people in admission for psychosis compared to the general population, with smaller elevations for other ethnic minority groups. Prevalence of schizophrenia in African and Caribbean countries is similar to Britain, while second generation Afro-Caribbean people have a higher risk than their parents, suggesting social not genetic reasons. David Bennett was an Afro-Caribbean schizophrenic man who suffocated while being restrained by four male nurses, leading to government acknowledgement of institutionalised racism in psychiatry. Hjern et al (2004) found schizophrenia risk ratios were levelled for ethnic minorities by adjusting for socioeconomic factors; elevated uncorrected ratios were also found amongst Finnish, Southern and Eastern European immigrants in Sweden.

Chinese and Indian racial subgroups in the UK do not have elevated rates of psychiatric admission for mental health issues (CHAI 2005), this may be due to different social conditions, different cultural concepts of mental health and different cross-cultural perception by medical staff. Loss of a mother before the age of 11 and looking after 3 or more children under the age of 14 were identified by Brown and Harris (1979) as major vulnerability factors for depression in adult women.

61 – J

Immersion in a fantasy world, combined with an introspective solitary outlook and indifference to praise or criticism suggests **schizoid personality disorder**. Art brut is created by people unrecognised by official culture, sometimes due to mental illness.

62 – C
Anxious (AKA avoidant) personality disorder leads to a preoccupation and hypersensitivity to rejection and a low self-image. Such people may avoid certain activities for fear of social rejection or disapproval

63 – F
People with **histrionic personality disorder** enjoy being the centre of attention. They tend to take great care of their appearance, with a tendency for exaggerated displays of emotion.

64 – A
Anankastic (ICD-10) **personality disorder** is termed obsessive-compulsive by DSM-IV. Such people crave a high degree of order, may be perfectionist to the detriment of social interaction, tend towards indecision and feel threatened by disruption.

65 – I
People with **paranoid personality disorder** tend to be litigious, stubborn, suspicious and sensitive in nature, with a tendency to take criticism personally. They may have elevated opinions of their talents, believing their potential to have been unfairly blighted.

Further Information (Q. 61 – 65)
ICD-10 classes personality disorders as developmental conditions rather than mental illness, below organic, drug-induced, psychotic, affective, anxiety-related and behavioural conditions in its diagnostic hierarchy. DSM-IV describes a personality disorder as "persistently inflexible and maladaptive personality traits, stable over time and which cause significant personal distress or functional impairment" and groups them into clusters A, B and C, with combined ~10% prevalence in the community.

Isolated traits of several personality disorders may be present without functional impairment or distress. Borderline personality disorder has ~2% prevalence (3:1 female predominance) with predisposition by abuse in childhood. Such people have difficulties forming stable close relationships due to an excessive fear of abandonment and an increased risk of self-harm. Opposition is mounting to UK government proposals making inpatient treatment of "dangerous severe personality disorders" compulsory, before any crime is committed, potentially indefinitely. Most criminals do not have personality disorders or mental illnesses, with major fraud and war crimes often perpetrated by "respectable" citizens.

Managing personality disorders involves social interventions, treating co-morbidities like substance abuse and a variety of psychological approaches such as cognitive behavioural and group therapy.

Cluster A – odd or eccentric
- Paranoid: feels others are plotting against them, suspicious of partners' fidelity, excessively self-important, bears grudges.
- Schizoid: solitary, does not seek close relationships, may have preoccupation with fantasy, indifferent to approval or criticism.

Cluster B – dramatic, erratic
- Antisocial and Borderline: see above.
- Impulsive: quarrelsome and volatile, may have trouble acting with long-term goals in mind.
- Histrionic: attention-seeking, exaggerated displays of emotion, inappropriate seductiveness, over-concern with physical attractiveness.
- Narcissistic: self-important, frequently high-achievers, crave admiration, may become aggressive when their self-image is challenged.

Cluster C – anxious, fearful
- Obsessive-compulsive (anankastic): excessive perfectionism, preoccupation with order, sticking rigidly to specific practices.
- Anxious/Avoidant: see above.
- Dependent: feel a need to be looked after, fearing being left to care for themselves, tending to allow others to make their decisions.

---

66 – J
This man has **mania** (as hinted by his **increased speech** and **reduced sleeping**) with psychosis, as witnessed by the grandiose **secondary delusion** that he controls the weather. A delusion of control (AKA delusion of passivity) is the fixed, unfounded and culturally inappropriate belief that outside forces are controlling you and is characteristic of schizophrenia.

67 – B
This is a **delusional memory**, in which **an imagined or genuine past event** is **given a new**, in this case persecutory, **interpretation**, suggesting a diagnosis of **schizophrenia**.

68 – I
This is a **delusion of thought withdrawal**, which is a first-rank symptom of **schizophrenia**.

69 – J
This is a secondary **delusion,** in this case of guilt, which has formed as a result of **psychotic depression**. This is always treated as severe.

70 – C
With a **delusional mood,** she feels something is afoot which they cannot explain. Delusional perceptions may subsequently arise to account for this unsettling state.

Further Information (Q. 66 – 70)
A delusion is a fixed and irrationally held belief that is incongruent with the patient's cultural background. Not all delusions are false, but the reasoning behind them makes no sense. Likewise, not all false and fixed beliefs are delusions, for example it is said that 50% of science taught at medical school will subsequently be proven factually wrong.

A **primary delusion** starts suddenly, without any abnormal event preceding it and is often a sign of schizophrenia. Delusions of mood, memory and perception are all primary delusions.

Secondary delusions occur following another abnormal psychiatric event, for example depression, hallucinations, or other delusions, forming a delusional system.

Folie a deux occurs when one deluded person influences another to share the same delusions. When they are separated, the person who acquired delusional beliefs normally loses them.

Nihilistic delusions are a form of secondary delusion seen in psychotic depression in which the person believes them, another person, or inanimate substances have ceased to exist. They may believe the World is ending, that they are dying, or that they have lost all their savings.

Delusions of control (a.k.a. delusions of passivity) occur when people believe they are being controlled by outside forces and strongly suggest schizophrenia, as do **delusions of perception** (a delusional interpretation is given to a real sensation), delusions of thought control (**insertion**- when it is felt that thoughts are placed inside by outside forces, **broadcast-** when thoughts are heard by others, **withdrawal-** when thoughts are removed) and persistent bizarre delusions. Delusional disorder features non-bizarre delusions in the absence of any other serious features, and hence cannot be classed as schizophrenia. Aside from their isolated delusion, the person may be quite highly-functioning.

---

71 – G

The overnight dexamethasone suppression test is a screening investigation for Cushing's disease; false positive results occur in up to 50% of people with severe depression (the 48-hour suppression test is more specific). Likewise, several studies have shown **subclinical hypothyroidism** occurring in depression (e.g. Bunevicius 1994). This can include mildly elevated TSH and attenuated TSH rise in response to TRH. **5-hydroxyindoleacetic acid (5-HIAA)** is a metabolite of **5-hydroxytryptamine (5-HT)**, levels of which are reduced in **depression**, according to the monoamine hypothesis. Several studies (e.g. Traskman et al (1981) found **reduced 5-HIAA in the cerebrospinal fluid (CSF) of suicide survivors**.

72 – C

Maternal rubella during gestation is associated with autism, the three main features of which this man displays.

73 – E

Damasio's somatic marker hypothesis (1995), proposes the orbitofrontal cortex (in the prefrontal) creates aversion to risk by inducing unpleasant autonomic associations (e.g. increased sweating), subconscious warning signs which constitute a "bad gut feeling". Damasio's Elliot was a patient who made impulsive misjudgments following his apparent recovery from a CVA that had bilaterally damaged his orbitofrontal cortex.

74 – D

He has a **delusion of perception**, which is a first-rank symptom of **schizophrenia**, and also displays negative features. Several studies have found increased lateral ventricle size (e.g. Weinberger and Wyatt 1982) with schizophrenia. Several other studies (see Powers 1999) have found atrophy or developmental abnormalities at other regions such as the **medial temporal lobes, lateral temporal cortex, prefrontal cortex**, many of which correlate the extent of the abnormality with the degree of negative schizophrenic symptoms. Verbal hallucinations have been correlated with elevated PET activity in the primary auditory cortex while thinking, which may cause internal voices to be perceived as external (Dierks et al 1997). **Elevated dopamine release** at the nucleus accumbens, of the **mesolimbic system**, is thought to be responsible for reward behaviour, whereby certain behaviours are neurologically incentivized by a pleasant feeling.-Massive dopamine release at the nucleus accumbens is caused by cocaine (which can also causes psychosis). Conventional reward behaviours such as eating and washing can be impaired in schizophrenia, but dysfunctional reward can act as a positive reinforcer when linked to delusions and hallucinations, or the compulsions of obsessive compulsive disorder and addiction (Carlson 2004).

75 – J
This scenario suggests Wernicke's encephalopathy, which is caused by vitamin B1 deficiency, seen in the West with chronic alcohol abuse, featuring **mamillary body atrophy** (located at the floor of the hypothalamus).

Further Information (Q. 71 – 75)
Raine et al (2000) found on imaging that people with **antisocial personality disorder** had an average **11% lower volume of grey matter in the prefrontal cortex**. Impaired prefrontal activity, either conditioned by childhood strife (e.g. indiscriminate punishment, no adverse associations made) or brain damage, is one hypothesis explaining antisocial personality disorder. However, a decreased volume of prefrontal grey matter is non-specific, and as SJ Gould wrote in "the Mismeasure of Man" (1996), Medicine has a long history of providing prejudiced biological explanations for societal ills

Silent lacunar infarcts have been associated with late-onset depression, Fujikawa et al (1993) found MRI evidence of silent CVA's in 66% of cases with onset over 65. CAG repeats on chromosome 4 are found with Huntington's chorea, an autosomal dominant condition leading to dementia, motor defects and possible emotional lability or depression. Inflammatory demyelination is a feature of multiple sclerosis, which can also lead to emotional lability and depression. Beta amyloid plaques and neurofibrillary tangles in the medial temporal lobes are a feature of Alzheimer's dementia.

The dopamine hypothesis of schizophrenia explained that positive symptoms were caused by dopamine excess in the mesolimbic pathway and negative symptoms by a lack of dopamine in the mesocortical pathway. Subsequent research suggests a more complicated aetiology.

The Dopamine Hypothesis

For	Against
- Levodopa (in Parkinson's patients) and other pro- dopaminergic drugs like cocaine, amphetamines, disulfiram (blocks dopamine breakdown) can induce positive symptoms of schizophrenia.	- Positive and negative symptoms of schizophrenia can be induced by ketamine or phencyclidine (PCP), which block NMDA glutamate receptors (Javitt and Zukin 1991). Other dopaminergic drugs like nicotine have no psychotic effects.
- Post-mortems of long-term schizophrenic patients show dopamine receptor up-regulation in the mesolimbic system.	- Post-mortems of long-term schizophrenic patients without medication history show no up-regulation, indicating it is drug-related and not causative.
- Efficacy of typical antipsychotics which are anti-dopaminergic (block D_2 receptor) have proven effects against positive symptoms, with Parkinsonian side-effects. Dopamine agonists like apomorphine can alleviate negative symptoms.	- Efficacy of atypical antipsychotics. These have limited affinity for D_2 receptors but are thought to work by blocking the $5HT_{2A}$ receptor. Unlike typical antipsychotics, they can alleviate positive and negative symptoms of the disease, with less risk of Parkinsonian side effects.
- Schizophrenic people release more dopamine in response to amphetamines than non-schizophrenics (Laruelle 1996).	- Aripiprazole, a partial dopamine agonist and atypical antipsychotic, is effective against positive and negative symptoms of schizophrenia.
- PCP infusion at prefrontal cortex increases dopamine release at the nucleus accumbens (Jentsch et al 1998)	

Weinberger et al (1988) proposed that reduced dorsolateral prefrontal activity caused negative and positive schizophrenia symptoms. Positive symptoms could occur through loss of inhibition transmitted by gabanergic connections from the dorsolateral prefrontal to the nucleus accumbens.

76 – F

Fregoli's syndrome is when a person deludedly believes strangers are people they know who have changed their appearance. It can be a result of schizophrenia, affective disorders and sometimes organic pathology such as right hemisphere damage.

77 – I

Features of **Wernicke-Korsakoff's syndrome** include **short-term memory loss, confabulation** (making up memories), **nystagmus, ataxia** and **abducens nerve (VI)** palsy. This is caused by **vitamin B1 deficiency**, occurring with malnutrition (beriberi) which may result from alcohol abuse.

It can also result from glucose infusions given without vitamins and other causes of damage to the mamillary bodies. Without early vitamin B1 replacement, Wernicke-Korsakoff's syndrome is irreversible, which is why IV multivitamins and glucose are often given to drunk patients with reduced consciousness.

78 – D

Cotard's syndrome consists of nihilistic delusions in depression. People with this syndrome may believe they have lost everything; they may think they are dead (hence cannot die), that their insides are rotting or that they have lost their life savings. This constitutes psychotic, and hence severe, depression.

79 – J

These are the **3 features of autism**. Asperger's does not feature a learning disability. Asperger's and autism are classed as pervasive developmental disorders, alongside Rett's syndrome and childhood disintegrative disorder.

80 – E

De Clerambault's syndrome AKA erotomania occurs when a person deludedly believes that someone (often famous) is in love with them, despite the absence of direct communication. This may lead to stalking and obsession.

Further Information (Q. 76 – 80)

Alice in Wonderland syndrome causes a subjective acceleration of time and is due to epilepsy or migraine.

Capgras syndrome occurs when a person believes that someone close to them has been replaced by an identical impostor. It can be caused by schizophrenia, affective disorders or organic disease like amygdala and right occipitotemporal damage. Hirstein and Ramachandran (1997) studied a man with Capgras syndrome; compared to normal controls, on seeing his mother, he lacked an increased galvanic sweat response (coordinated by the amygdala) compared to when he saw strangers. However, this was intact when he heard her voice on the phone, whereupon he would recognise her.

Munchausen's syndrome is a controversial condition describing individuals who feign symptoms, often to obtain unnecessary medical treatment.

Tourette's syndrome is characterized by impaired impulse control, featuring compulsive vocal and motor tics and associated with obsessive compulsive disorder. People with Tourette's can uncontrollably cry out offensive language, which becomes grunts and growls as they try to muffle themselves.

---

81 – D
The key features are the **marco-orchidism** and **large ears**, which suggest **Fragile X syndrome**, the **2nd commonest form of learning disability**. It stems from CGG triplet repeats on the X chromosome's long arm, affecting 0.5-1 per 1000 males and ~1 per 2000 females. Female carriers of the gene have learning disabilities in ~1/3 of cases and it is **associated with autism**.

82 – C
Fetal alcohol syndrome is suggested by learning disabilities with **small stature, small eyes and facial malformations.** Pregnant women are advised not to drink, especially in the first trimester.

83 – I
Rubella embryopathy is suggested particularly by **congenital cataracts** and can seriously damage the foetus, especially in the first trimester. Other features include deafness, small eyes, hydrocephalus, microcephaly and learning disabilities (may feature autism). If MMR vaccination rates remain dangerously low in the UK, more cases of rubella embryopathy are likely to be seen.

84 – B

These are 2 characteristics of **Down syndrome**, the **commonest cause of learning disability in the UK**.

Other features that might be mentioned in EMQs include high arch palate, hyperextensible joints, iris (Brushfield's) spots, congenital cardiac (atrio-ventricular septal defect) and gastrointestinal defects (duodenal atresia), increased risk of leukaemia and early-onset Alzheimer's. Life expectancy is ~50 years. It is due to a trisomy or translocation at chromosome 21. Effects are less severe with tissue mosaicism, whereby the mutation occurs in the developing embryo and only a proportion of cells are affected.

The **major risk factor** is **maternal age**, with a risk of 1/2000 at age 20, 1/365 at 35, 1/110 at 40 and 1/30 at 45, with an overall rate of 1.5/1000 live births. Antenatal screening includes ultrasound for fetal nuchal translucency and defects, human chorionic gonadotrophin (raised in Down syndrome), inhibin A (raised), pregnancy associated plasma protein A (reduced), oestriol (reduced), maternal blood tests like alpha-fetoprotein (raised by neural tube defects, reduced in Down syndrome), with definitive diagnosis by invasive tests such as chorionic villus sampling or amniocentesis, each of which have a small risk of inducing miscarriage.

85 – H

The key feature is the **regression of development markers**, suggesting **Rett's syndrome** (a type of pervasive developmental disorder) which **affects girls almost exclusively** (~4/10 000 female births) leading to profound learning and physical disabilities. Head growth decelerates, with loss of purposeful hand movements and speech.

Further Information (Q. 81 – 85)

Prader-Willi syndrome affects 1 child per 25 000, causing learning disabilities, overeating and hypogonadism. Tuberous sclerosis is a rare autosomal dominant disorder that can cause nodules to grow in the skin, brain, spleen, kidney, lungs and retina. This can lead to epilepsy but has variable penetrance, causing learning disabilities in up to 70% of cases. Phenylketonuria is an autosomal recessive inherited condition occurring in ~1 per 15000 births whereby phenylalanine hydroxylase deficiency leads to impaired metabolism of phenylalanine and learning disability. This can be prevented if a diet low in phenylalanine and rich in tyrosine is followed for life; newborns in the UK are screened.

Severity	Prevalence	IQ range	Clinical features
Mild	3% (males predominate)	50-69	Most can work and live independently. Language development delayed, may have literacy problems and be particularly vulnerable to manipulation.
Moderate	0.15%	35-49	Limited language development, most are not fully independent, and may work with supervision.
Severe	0.15%	20-34	Likely to have some physical disability. Language is very limited. Not independent.
Profound	0.05%	<20	Likely to have severe physical disability, are often incontinent. May not have any language skills. Require supervision and care. May learn some new skills but only very slowly.

Note that intelligence comes in many forms and testing was developed by Alfred Binet purely to identify special educational needs (see SJ Gould's "Mismeasure of Man" for the hidden agendas that later developed in biometrics). Learning disability is defined by the WHO ICD-10 classification as a "condition of arrested or incomplete development of the mind" characterised by significant impairment of social or adaptive functioning and significant global impairment of intelligence that arose during the developmental period. Mental illness in people with learning disabilities is more common than in the general population. It can be difficult to diagnose due to differing presentation. For example, biological symptoms of depression like loss of appetite and sleep disturbance may be of more relevant to diagnosis than mood change.

86 – B

Antifreeze contains **ethylene glycol**, the metabolism of which is increased by **alcohol**. Ethylene glycol poisoning can also be treated with peritoneal dialysis.

87 – I

Naloxone is an **opiate antagonist** used for treatment of heroin overdose which rapidly reverses opiate actions, causing pain and diarrhoea. However, it is **rapidly metabolised**, necessitating monitoring and repeated injections. Methadone and dextropropoxyphene are opiates with longer half-lives than heroin and overdose requires extended naloxone therapy, perhaps by IV infusion.

88 – H

N-acetylcysteine is the **antidote for paracetamol** overdose; his symptoms suggest severe poisoning. Fatal paracetamol overdoses can be initially asymptomatic, causing death by acute liver failure days later. The decision to treat with N-acetylcysteine is made by monitoring blood paracetamol concentration and comparing to the drug treatment line, with consideration for markers of severe poisoning such as HIV positivity, large overdoses, hyperbilirubinaemia and abnormal liver function tests within 12 hours.

89 – E

Disulfiram inhibits metabolism of alcohol at the liver so that ingesting small amounts of alcohol, even in medicines or mouthwashes, causes accumulation of acetaldehyde, leading to headaches, nausea, tachycardia and palpitations. Larger amounts can cause arrhythmias and collapse. Patients should be alcohol-free for at least 24 hours before starting treatment, which should only be under specialist supervision. Continuation of treatment is determined solely by patient self-motivation. As a P450 enzyme inhibitor, disulfiram slows breakdown of liver-metabolised drugs like warfarin and phenytoin. Naltrexone can be given to maintain abstinence from alcohol use or reduce severity of relapse, but at the time of writing was not licensed in the UK for this application.

90 – J

As she is no longer dependent on heroin, methadone, an opiate agonist, is not desirable. **Naltrexone**, a partial **opiate antagonist**, used to prevent relapse in heroin (when opioid free for minimum of 7 days) and alcohol addiction; it blocks enjoyment of drug abuse and reduces withdrawal symptoms.

Further Information (Q. 86 – 90)

Initial measures in the treatment of poisoning include maintaining an open airway and maintaining circulation, possible by IV fluids. History-taking and analysis of the scene may reveal the poison ingested, with further information provided by serum and urine drug screens, LFT's, blood glucose, ABG, U&E and clotting studies.

Poison	Remedy	Poison	Remedy
Aspirin	Activated charcoal	Ethylene glycol	Alcohol
Benzodiazepines	Flumazenil	Heroin	Naloxone
Beta blockers	Atropine	Iron	Desferrioxamine chelation, haemodialysis
Carbon monoxide	100% oxygen	Lithium	Haemodialysis
Cyanide	Dicobolt editate, amyl nitrite	Methanol, Ethanol	Haemodialysis, vitamins, glucose
Digoxin	Digoxin antibody fragments	Paracetamol	N-Acetyl cysteine

Activated charcoal is used to adsorb poisons from the stomach. However, it is no use 1 hour after ingestion because the stomach empties, apart from with poisons that reduce gastric motility such as tricyclic antidepressants and aspirin. Multiple-dose activated charcoal may be used to prevent absorption from the gut, following life-threatening overdoses with aspirin, carbamazepine, dapsone, phenobarbitone, quinine and theophylline. Buprenorphine is a partial opioid agonist used to treat moderate opioid dependence. When in doubt with regard to appropriate treatment, it is recommended to consult a poisons information centre.

91 – E
Borderline personality disorder is **~3 times more common in women** than men. Its overall prevalence is **~2%**.

92 – C
From 2004-2007, the average UK prison suicide incidence was **101 per 100,000** per year (Ministry of Justice 2008), while the 2006 rate amongst the general public was 11.4 (Office for National Statistics). However, in 2008, it was reported that the number taking their lives fell to 61, at a rate of 91 per 100,000. Non-fatal self-harm is particularly common amongst women prisoners.

93 – D
There is **no difference from the UK lifetime prevalence** (Cooper 2005). The increased rate of schizophrenia amongst immigrants and their offspring is due to **social** not genetic factors.

94 – D
This is **equal to the male predisposition**.

95 – H
The **daily safe limit** for **males** is **4 units**, with a maximum weekly total of 21 units. For **women**, the daily limit is **3 units**, with a maximum weekly total of 14 units (1 unit= 8g or 10ml of ethanol). The Office for National statistics (2006) reported that **35% of UK men questioned exceeded the daily limit** for at least one day in the previous week, compared to 20% amongst women.

Further Information (Q. 91 – 95)

Disorder	Mean UK lifetime prevalence (all vary with social class, region, race etc)
Schizophrenia	~1%
Recurrent depressive disorder	10-25% in females, 5-12% in males
Bipolar disorder	~1%
Generalised anxiety disorder	10-20%
Borderline personality disorder	~2%

96 – J
The **police** have deemed this patient in need of **care and control** in a public place and can detain her to a place of safety for **72 hours** under **section 136**.

97 – D
First-level trained nurses can apply **section 5(4)** and it lasts **6 hours**.

98 – B
Section 3 is a compulsory admission for treatment, applied for by an **approved social worker** or the **patient's nearest relative**.

99 – I
This irreversible and potentially dangerous procedure would require a **section 59**. This means that the **patient must give informed consent** and **approval must be given by a doctor from a separate team**. Less radical procedures such as electro-convulsive therapy can be given to patients under section 58 with valid consent or approval from a second

independent doctor, though in the case of a life-threatening emergency, under section 62 neither are required.

100 – F
Section 37 is used to send mentally ill offenders to compulsory inpatient psychiatric treatment.

Further Information (Q. 96 – 100)
For summary of sections 2-5(4) see OSCE question 14.

Mental Health Act 1983 (amended 2007) Part III. Patients concerned in criminal proceedings or under sentence
These sections require recommendations from 2 doctors, not necessarily from separate hospitals and the decision is made by a magistrate or judge. Approved social workers and nearest relatives have no say. However, they can only be carried out if the hospital representatives can guarantee to make a bed available within a certain time limit.

Section 35 – remand to hospital for assessment. This is made prior to trial when the accused is suspected of being mentally ill. It is based on the recommendation of at least one doctor and lasts 28 days, extendable up to 12 weeks. The order allows assessment but no treatment and the accused must be admitted within 7 days. They can only be discharged with further court involvement.

Section 36 – enables compulsory admission for treatment after conviction but before sentencing.

Section 37 – hospital order. A mentally ill offender may be detained for compulsory treatment in a psychiatric hospital instead of prison based on the recommendation of 2 doctors, one of whom must be section 12 approved. This lasts at least 6 months with no right of appeal during this period and can subsequently be extended.

Section 48 – enables emergency transfer of pre-trial prisoners to hospital for treatment, by Home Office warrant, requires recommendation from 2 doctors.

6   Introduction to OSCEs

SETUP

OSCE stands for "Objective Specific Clinical Examination". Exams may contain up to 25 OSCE stations, each lasting 5 to 10 minutes. OSCEs may test history-taking, examination, communication, written and diagnostic skills, involving professional actors or actual patients. In some cases, written material may be provided, which you would typically be given 5 minutes to read.

There follow 40 OSCEs (20 for neurology and 20 for psychiatry) with full mark schemes, together with actor briefs for the patient (which can be played by a friend). Although the marks given in each scheme vary, for the final mark each station counts equally i.e. getting 20/20 in one station counts the same as getting 40/40 for another.

To replicate exam conditions, we have also included additional viva questions which examiners may ask at the end of the session. These are often used to identify the top students.

In some cases, the examiners may make up viva questions on the spot (as opposed to using prepared questions). They would then engage in a discussion with you on the answer that you have provided. It therefore makes sense to steer the discussion in a direction that suits you. For example, if asked to give a list of conditions causing peripheral neuropathy, you would aim to list the conditions that you feel comfortable talking at greater length about.

COMMON POINTS

There are aspects of a candidate's performance which examiners would expect to find in all OSCEs. These include polite introductions, checking the patient's identity, asking about pain and washing your hands before examining a patient, and thanking them where appropriate. In explanation stations, it is important to assess the patient's prior level of knowledge, check their understanding of what you have said, ask for questions and offer written information. A common trick is for the examiner to keep patient information leaflets hidden until the candidate mentions them. In the history stations, summarising what you understand they have said, then politely asking "what else would you like to add?" and "do you have any questions for me?" if your mind goes blank, can help.

CLINICAL EXAMINATION

When tested on clinical examination in medical finals, genuine patients with real signs are often present. When examining the volunteer, you only need address the examiner to mention painful tests that you are not going to perform but would consider in real practice.The onus is on the candidate to demonstrate a methodical examination, uncovering the major signs in the limited time available. Therefore, giving a running commentary of your actions is rarely useful as it slows you down and is distracting. There is little to gain by listing signs you are looking for; if you notice a sign on inspection, mention it in your presentation. However, make sure to clearly demonstrate inspection from the end of the bed and from close up.

All stations will have an <u>automatic fail</u> for being rude or unsafe; it helps to call patients "sir", "madam", or their real name preceded by Mr/Mrs/Ms. Before touching patients, check that they have no pain and before repositioning them or making them walk, ask if they are comfortable and steady doing this. If you do accidentally cause pain, it is best to apologise and proceed carefully.

Early on, take a step back to inspect the exposed patient, noting pointers like a wheelchair by the bed or characteristic skin lesions. Ask the patient to walk if they are able, because gaits can be characteristic. You should look for key signs as a clinical picture forms e.g. tongue fasciculation in suspected motor neurone disease. You should be able to present your findings in about 30 seconds. It helps to practise describing examination findings of "textbook" (i.e. featuring all the distinctive signs, not necessarily like in real life) cases e.g. for multiple sclerosis:

"I examined a middle-aged man who was comfortable at rest. On inspection, he was fitted with a urinary catheter and had pronator drift. He used two walking sticks and had scissor gait. Tone was increased, with clasp knife reflex in his arms and clonus in both ankles. Power was reduced bilaterally, scoring 4 out of 5, and was more impaired in the legs. Biceps,

triceps, supinator, knee and ankle jerk reflexes were exaggerated; Babinski's reflex was present bilaterally. Nociception, vibroception, proprioception and light touch sense were impaired in both legs. Coordination was impaired, partly due to muscle weakness. On flexion of the neck, L'Hermitte's sign was present. There was no tremor, fasciculation (including tongue) or other uncontrolled movements at rest. To complete my examination I would like to test cranial nerve function including for relative afferent papillary defect, diplopia and nystagmus, and take a full history. My primary diagnosis is multiple sclerosis, differentials include cervical cord compression, cerebral palsy, myelitis, bilateral CVA and motor neurone disease."

QUESTION STYLES

In OSCEs (as in real-life history-taking), it is important to let the patient do most of the talking. Furthermore, patients will give more information when asked open-ended questions e.g. "How does this affect your life?" and "Tell me more about that." Although many of the scripts are arranged in response to specific cues, asking open questions will cause the actors to lead you in the correct direction, or even go into cued parts of their history when given the chance.

However, there are instances, such as with diagnosis of cauda equina syndrome and epilepsy when specific issues such as sexual function, bladder and bowel control have to be raised, as the patient would be reluctant to mention them initially. In the diagnosis of emergencies such as meningitis, the scenarios focus on prioritising key features in the history, including blanching or non-blanching rash, cold peripheries, joint pain and neck stiffness, which requires specific closed questions. Weight loss is a marker of serious organic and psychiatric illness and should not be missed.

When considering the cause of a disease, a surgical sieve mnemonic may help, such as "**INVITE MItCH Down**", standing for Infection, **N**eoplasm, **V**ascular, auto**I**mmune, **T**rauma, **E**ndocrine, **M**etabolic, **I**diopathic, **C**ongenital, **H**aematological, **D**rug-related, **D**egenerative.

HISTORY STRUCTURE

This should include the presenting complaint, history of presenting complaint, past medical, surgical and psychiatric history, drug history and allergies, family history, social history and systems review, though in these five minute stations, only more truncated histories can be obtained.

The components of a psychiatric mental state examination can be remembered as:

- **ABC** (**A**ppearance, **B**ehaviour, **C**ognition),
- **RST** (**R**apport, **S**peech, **T**hought pattern),
- **IMP** (**I**nsight, **M**ood, **P**erception).

The psychiatric OSCEs are drafted to the ICD-10 (the World Health Organisation's International Classification of Diseases) hierarchical system, whereby organic and drug-induced conditions have to be excluded before a psychiatric illness can be diagnosed, with first consideration given to psychotic, followed by affective, somatoform (anxiety-related), behavioural syndromes (e.g. anorexia nervosa, sleep disorders), personality disorders, mental retardation, psychological developmental disorders, then childhood behavioural and emotional syndromes.

Conditions not fitting into these criteria are classed as unspecified mental illness. Diseases higher up in the hierarchy can cause the diagnostic criteria of disorders lower down (e.g. alcohol addiction causing depression), though doctors are advised to make as many diagnoses in a patient as they think necessary to fully describe the complexity of their condition.

By the DSM-IV classification (Diagnostic and Statistical Manual of mental disorders), followed in the US, the patient is diagnosed with all the conditions for which they fulfil the criteria, regardless of their position on the hierarchy. This allows for more prescriptions to be made, incentivising the diagnosis of more recently recognised (and potentially lucrative) conditions like attention deficit hyperactivity disorder.

7   Neurology OSCEs

OSCE 1 – Examination [5 minutes]
(See page 124 for actor's brief and marking scheme)

Perform a neurological examination of the upper limbs of this patient, explaining to the examiner as you go along but omitting painful tests. Answer the examiner's questions at the end:

Provided: tendon hammer, cotton wool, 128 Hz tuning fork, alcohol handrub.

OSCE 2 – Examination [5 minutes]
(See page 126 for actor's brief and marking scheme)

Perform a neurological examination of the lower limbs of this patient, explaining to the examiner as you go along but omitting painful tests. Answer the examiner's questions at the end

Provided: tendon hammer, cotton wool, orange stick, 128 Hz tuning fork, alcohol handrub.

OSCE 3 – History [5 minutes]
(See page 131 for actor's brief and marking scheme)

You are working for an out-of-hours service when you receive a telephone call from a concerned mother. Take a history from her with a view to making a diagnosis and answer the examiner's questions.

OSCE 4 – History [5 minutes]
(See page 135 for actor's brief and marking scheme)

You are a medical student in Accident and Emergency. Please take a history from a 64-year-old woman who has a headache, with a view to making a diagnosis and answer the examiner's questions at the end.

OSCE 5 – History [5 minutes]
(See page 138 for actor's brief and marking scheme)

You are a medical student at a general practice. Please take a history from Beth Garner, a 35-year-old woman who complains of tiredness, with a view to making a diagnosis.

OSCE 6 – History [5 minutes]
(See page 141 for actor's brief and marking scheme)

You are a medical student at a general practice. Please take a history from a 38-year-old man with back pain, with a view to making a diagnosis.

OSCE 7 – Examination [5 minutes]
(See page 145 for actor's brief and marking scheme)

Perform fundoscopy and acuity testing on this model, addressing the examiner as the patient and answering their questions at the end.

Provided: eye model, visual acuity chart, fundoscope.

OSCE 8 – History [5 minutes]
(See page 148 for actor's brief and marking scheme)

You are a medical student at a general practice. Please take a history from a 40-year-old woman in pain, with a view to making a diagnosis. The examiner will ask you some questions near the end.

OSCE 9 – History [5 minutes]
(See page 151 for actor's brief and marking scheme)

You are a medical student at a general practice. Please take a history from a 27-year-old woman who has tingling in her hand, with a view to making a diagnosis. The examiner will ask you some questions near the end.

OSCE 10 – Written station: investigations [5 minutes]
(See page 154 for answers and explanations)

Read the results and match the correct diagnosis from the options below.

A Absence seizure
B Carpal tunnel syndrome
C Lambert-Eaton syndrome
D Mononeuritis multiplex
E Motor neurone disease

F Myasthenia gravis
G Myotonia
H Nerve root avulsion
I Tonic clonic seizure
J Tonic seizure

1. Edrophonium injection causes definite alleviation of muscle weakness within 1 minute.

2. Electromyelogram traces of the tongue find fibrillation potentials, of maximum amplitude 200 microvolts.

3. Electromyelogram shows waxing and waning frequency of muscle potentials.

4. Electroencephalogram shows 3Hz bilateral symmetrical spike and wave activity when the patient hyperventilates.

5. Electroencephalogram shows widespread 10Hz signal during a seizure.

6. Electroencephalogram shows widespread 10Hz signal which progresses to a mixture of slow waves and spikes.

7. Nerve conduction testing shows normal sensory action potentials in a patient's numb right arm following a car crash.

8. Nerve conduction study shows delayed transmission at the ulnar nerve in the upper left arm and the median nerve in the right forearm.

9. Nerve conduction study show transiently increased amplitude of muscular response on repeated stimulation.

10. Nerve conduction study shows delayed transmission in the median nerve across the wrist.

OSCE 11 – Written station: Neuroimaging [5 minutes]
(See page 157 for answers and explanations)

For each scenario, match the correct diagnosis from the options below

A Cerebral abscess
B Cerebral metastasis
C Cerebrovascular accident
D Extradural haemorrhage
E Glioma

F Meningioma
G Multiple sclerosis
H Neurocysticercosis
I Sarcoidosis
J Subdural haemorrhage

1. MRI T2-weighted image shows periventricular high signal lesions which enhance with gadolinium-DTPA, causing sunray appearance on sagittal view.

2. CT scan shows biconvex high density lesion bordering right parietal and temporal bones.

3. CT scan shows wedge-shaped lesion of reduced density bordering right occipital bone and extending towards lateral ventricle.

4. MRI T1-weighed coronal image shows round isodense lesion that uniformly enhances with gadolinium-DTPA, bordering the tentorium cerebelli.

5. MRI T1-weighted coronal image shows ring-enhancing lesion in the right parietal lobe with surrounding area of reduced intensity.

6. CT scan shows multiple small areas of increased density, though MRI scan is normal.

7. CT scan shows a low-density lesion in the frontal lobe that enhances irregularly with iodine, causing deviation of the midline and contraction of the lateral ventricles.

8. MRI T1-weighted image shows 20 small round lesions that enhance with gadolinium.

9. CT scan shows a crescent-shaped low density area bordering the right parietal bone.

10. CT scan shows 2 enhancing lesions in the left frontal and right parietal lobes, each with surrounding areas of low density.

OSCE 12 – Explaining Alzheimer's disease [5 minutes]
(See page 160 for actor's brief and marking scheme)

Mrs Rita Edmonds, 55, has a mother recently diagnosed with Alzheimer's disease at the age of 82. On investigation, she had normal serum levels of vitamin B12, and folic acid, normal urine and normal thyroid function, plus negative syphilis serology; the diagnosis was based on memory assessment by the GP, clinical history and examination. She is being seen at a memory clinic to evaluate whether she is suitable for drug therapy and if she needs further investigation. Discuss the illness with her.

OSCE 13 – Epilepsy advice [5 minutes]
(See page 163 for actor's brief and marking scheme)

Ms Jennifer White, 18, has recently been diagnosed with idiopathic epilepsy and has suffered several tonic-clonic seizures. She is being treated with carbamazepine. Advise her on how it will affect her life.

OSCE 14 – History [5 minutes]
(See page 166 for actor's brief and marking scheme)

You are a medical student at a general practice. Please take a history from a 41-year-old woman with a headache.

OSCE 15 – History [5 minutes]
(See page 170 for actor's brief and marking scheme)

You are a medical student at a neurology outpatients' clinic. Please take a history from a 16-year-old boy who has had some unusual episodes, with a view to making a diagnosis.

OSCE 16 – History [5 minutes]
(See page 174 for actor's brief and marking scheme)

You are a medical student at an accident and emergency department. Please take a history from a 19-year-old woman with a severe headache and answer the examiner's questions at the end.

OSCE 17 – History [5 minutes]
(See page 177 for actor's brief and marking scheme)

You are a medical student at a general practice. Please take a history from a 31-year-old woman with headaches with a view to making a diagnosis. The examiner will ask some questions near the end.

OSCE 18 – Consent for lumbar puncture [5 minutes]
(See page 181 for actor's brief and marking scheme)

Tariq Achebe, 22, has suspected bacterial meningitis. He has been started on antibiotics, his CT scan was normal and lumbar puncture is planned. Explain the procedure to him with a view to obtaining informed consent.

OSCE 19 – History [5 minutes]
(See page 183 for actor's brief and marking scheme)

You are a medical student at a GP's surgery; please take a history from Marcus Redding, 24, who has inflamed eyes, with a view to making a diagnosis.

OSCE 20 – Examination [10 minutes]
(See page 186 for actor's brief and marking scheme)

Examine the cranial nerves of this patient in their correct order. Fundoscopy and otoscopy are not required, mention – but do not perform – any uncomfortable tests.

Be prepared to move on at the examiner's discretion and answer their questions at the end.

Provided: pen torch, cotton wool, tendon hammer, Snellen chart, 256 Hz tuning fork, alcohol handrub

8 Neurology OSCEs Actor's brief & marking scheme

OSCE 1 – Examination

Marking Scheme	
2 marks: Good - 1 mark: Adequate - 0 mark: Poor/Not done	**Mark 0 – 2**
1. Polite introduction, explains what they will do, gains consent.	☐
2. Washes their hands.	☐
3. Asks about pain before touching.	☐
4. Looks around the bed for Zimmer frames, catheters etc. Comments on appearance.	☐
5. Exposes upper limbs, looks for posture, asymmetry, wasting, tremor, fasciculation, neurofibromas etc.	☐
6. Tests for pronator drift: asks patient to hold both arms out with palms pointing up & eyes shut (slow pronation indicates UMN)	☐
7. Observes for resting tremor.	☐
8. Tone: passive movement at shoulder, elbow and wrist.	☐
9. Power: ▪ shoulder abduction (C5-6), adduction (C6-8)	☐
10. ▪ elbow flexion (C5-6), extension (C7-8)	☐
11. ▪ wrist flexion (C6-7), extension (C7-8), grip (C7-8)	☐
12. ▪ thumb opposition (median nerve), thumb abduction (radial nerve), finger abduction and adduction (ulnar nerve)	☐
13. Reflexes: ▪ biceps jerk (C5-6)	☐
14. ▪ triceps jerk (C7-8)	☐
15. ▪ supinator jerk (C5-6)	☐
16. ▪ finger jerk (C8)	☐
17. Explains that they would test for nociception, starting peripherally.	☐
18. Tests for vibration sense using 128 Hz tuning fork, starting on fingertips, working proximally if not felt.	☐

19. Tests for temperature sense using tuning fork. □
    "Does this feel hot or cold?"
20. Tests for proprioception with sufficiently small increments, □
    starting peripherally and moving proximally if not detected.
21. Tests for fine touch with cotton wool, demonstrating □
    knowledge of dermatomes.
22. Co-ordination: asks to touch their nose with either index □
    finger. Asks to touch index fingers together with eyes shut
    (Yasen's test).
23. Tests for dysdiadochokinesis: one hand on top of the other, □
    asks patient to rotate palm up and down as quickly as they
    can.
24. Tests for function e.g. undoing a button. □
25. Thanks the patient; covers them up. Overall impression. □

Examiner's additional questions

Q: **What posture would you expect in a person with a
left middle cerebral artery cerebrovascular accident?**
26. A: Right arm flexed, right leg extended. □

Q: **Give some causes of combined upper and lower
motor neurone signs.**
27. A: Spinal cord lesion causing LMN at level of damage and □
    UMN below, severe vitamin B12 deficiency causing subacute
    combined spinal cord degeneration, dual pathology (e.g.
    CVA and diabetic neuropathy), motor neurone disease.

TOTAL SCORE | **/ 54**

OSCE 2 – Examination

Marking Scheme	
2 marks: Good - 1 mark: Adequate - 0 mark: Poor/Not done	**Mark 0 – 2**

1. Polite introduction, explains what they will do, gains consent. ☐
2. Washes their hands. ☐
3. Asks about pain before touching. ☐
4. Looks around bed for Zimmer frame, walking stick, urinary catheter etc. ☐
5. Tests walking, checking this is safe for them. Looks for specific gaits, e.g. broad-based (cerebellar), stamping (sensory neuropathy), shuffling (Parkinsonian), scissor (UMN), foot drop (motor neuropathy), etc. ☐
6. Exposes lower limbs, and looks for posture, asymmetry, wasting, and fasciculation etc, comments on appearance. ☐
7. Tone: ▪ Passive movement at hips, knees and ankle ☐
8. ▪ Tests for patellar and ankle clonus ☐
9. Power: ▪ Hip flexion (L2,3), extension (L5, S1,2) ☐
10. ▪ Knee flexion (L5,S1), extension (L3,4) ☐
11. ▪ Ankle dorsiflexion (L4,5), plantar flexion (S1,2) ☐
12. Reflexes ▪ Knee jerk (L3,4) ☐
13. ▪ Ankle jerk (L4,5) ☐
14. ▪ Plantar reflex (L5, S1, S2) ☐
15. Explains that they would test for nociception, starting peripherally. ☐
16. Tests for vibration sense using 128 Hz tuning fork, starting on fingertips, working proximally if not felt. ☐
17. Tests for temperature sense using tuning fork. "Does this feel hot or cold?" ☐
18. Tests proprioception by small increments, toe not touching adjacent skin. Starts peripherally and moves proximally if impaired. ☐
19. Tests for fine touch with cotton wool, demonstrating knowledge of dermatomes. ☐
20. Co-ordination: asks to rub heel up shin, on either side, toe pointing (looking for intention tremor). ☐
21. Thanks the patient; covers them up. Overall impression. ☐

Examiner's additional questions

Q: **Give some causes of peripheral neuropathy.**

22. **A:** Alcohol abuse, vitamin B12 deficiency, cancer, drugs (e.g. methotrexate, diabetic neuropathy, Charcot-Marie-Tooth disease). ☐

Q: **What is Brown-Séquard syndrome?**

23. **A:** Brown-Séquard syndrome: hemisection of spine causing UMN lesion ipsilateral and below, LMN at level ipsilaterally, vibroception, fine touch and proprioception loss ipsilateral and below, pain and temperature loss contralateral and below. ☐

TOTAL SCORE | **/ 46**

Further information (OSCEs 1 & 2)

The components of neurological examination can be remembered as **ATP RSC** – **A**ppearance, **T**one, **P**ower, **R**eflexes, **S**ensation, Co-ordination (Eves 2004).

Pyramidal lesions affect the corticospinal tract, and are classed as **lower motor neurone (LMN)** or **upper motor neurone (UMN)**. UMN lesions result from damage between the motor cortex and synapses at the ventral horn. LMN lesions result from damage between the ventral roots and neuromuscular junction. **Clasp knife rigidity** occurs with UMN lesion; the limb resists passive movement, and then suddenly gives way. **Clonus** is also seen with UMN- rapid passive stretches (e.g. ankle dorsiflexion, stretching the gastrocnemius) cause bursts of muscle contractions. Extensor plantar response (**Babinski**), with upwards deviation of the big toe and fanning of the others is abnormal in adults and occurs with UMN injury, coma or after a generalised seizure (Jackson's paresis). Power should be tested after active movement has been demonstrated.

Apical lung cancer may cause Horner's syndrome (cervical sympathetic damage) and C8-T2 radiculopathy, featuring arm pain and wasting of the small muscles of the hand (Pancoast syndrome). Mixed UMN and LMN signs (e.g. upwards plantar reflex, absent ankle jerk) can be caused by dual pathology (e.g. CVA and peripheral neuropathy), conditions like motor neuron disease or conus medullaris damage, (UMN/LMN junction affected), severe B12 deficiency causing peripheral neuropathy (e.g. absent ankle jerk) and subacute degeneration of the spinal cord (e.g. upward plantars and exaggerated knee jerk), syphilitic taboparesis, multisystem degeneration (e.g. Friedrich's ataxia). Extra-pyramidal lesions do not follow the same pattern because they do not affect the corticospinal tract.

The cerebellum is involved in balance and coordination, while basal ganglia functions include basic motor control and stimulus-response memory. Yasen's sign occurs with cerebellar damage and is being unable bring the index fingers together tip-to-tip with the eyes closed. Parkinsonian lesions (basal ganglia affected) hinder initiation and cessation of deliberate movement. Balance is poor and a wheeled Zimmer frame may be seen at the bedside. Cogwheel rigidity occurs when the forearm is passively supinated in incremental rhythmic jerks due to resting tremor causing fluctuating resistance. Lead pipe rigidity is seen in more advanced disease, with unvaryingly stiff limbs.

Cerebellar signs can be remembered by the mnemonic **DANISH**-
Dysdiadochokinesis, **A**taxia, **N**ystagmus, **I**ntention tremor, **S**lurred or **S**taccato speech (cannot enunciate "British Constitution"), **H**ypotonia.

Parkinsonian signs can be remembered as **TRAPS**: resting **T**remor, **R**igidity, **A**kinesia, **P**ostural instability, **S**huffling gait.

Motor lesion: Pyramidal

	Upper motor neurone lesion	Lower motor neurone lesion
Appearance	No early wasting, pronator drift, CVA causes flexed arm & extended leg posture (anti-gravity muscles relatively spared), bilateral spinal cord damage may cause scissor gait (hips and knees slightly flexed, legs crossed)	Early wasting, fasciculation, high stepping gait may be seen with foot-drop.
Tone	Increased, clasp knife rigidity and clonus may be present.	Reduced.
Power	Reduced	Reduced
Reflex	Exaggerated, Babinski plantar reflex (big toe points up).	Reduced.
Coordination	Reduced	Reduced
Examples	CVA, motor neuron disease, spinal cord injury, multiple sclerosis, space occupying lesion.	Peripheral neuropathy, Guillain-Barré syndrome, motor neurone disease, cauda equina syndrome.

Motor lesion: Extra-Pyramidal

	Cerebellar lesions	Parkinsonian
Appearance	No wasting. Broad-based gait. Intention tremor.	No wasting, festinant (shuffling) stooped gait with little armswing, freezing/akinesia, greasy skin, sialorrhoea, mask-like face (hypomimetic), resting tremor.
Tone	Reduced.	Increased- lead pipe or cogwheeling
Power	Not affected.	Not affected.
Reflex	Not diminished or increased. May have pendular knee jerk.	Not affected.
Co-ordination	Reduced. Balance problems. Yasen's sign. Dysdiadochokinesis.	Reduced. Balance problems.
Other	Slurred speech, nystagmus.	Micrographia (small writing)
Examples	Cerebellar stroke, progressive multifocal leucoencephalopathy, tumour, benign essential tremor, alcohol toxicity, cerebellar abscess.	Idiopathic (Parkinson's disease), drug-induced (anti-dopamine drugs, MPTP), post-sleeping sickness

Sensory testing consists of dorsal column (proprioception, vibration sense, fine touch) and spinothalamic modalities (pain, crude touch and temperature). In an OSCE, pain generally is not tested, but it should be mentioned. Dermatomes vary between people but can be approximated as follows:

C5-6: shoulders, upper arm, radial forearm, thumb and index finger.
C7: middle finger.
C8: other fingers and ulnar forearm.   **T1**: armpit.
T4: nipples.   **T10**: navel.
L1: inguinal ligament area.   **L2**: anterior upper thigh.
L3: front of knee.   **L4**: medial lower leg.
L5: lateral lower leg, medial foot dorsum to big toe.
S1: heel and sole.   **S2**: back of thigh.
S3-5: anus and anal canal.

On the palm, the median nerve provides sensory innervation of the thumb, middle finger, index finger, half the ring finger and the adjoining palm. This region is painful in **carpal tunnel syndrome**. The ulnar nerve supplies the ulnar one and a half fingers. On the dorsum, the median nerve supplies only the distal phalanges of the same 3 and a half fingers, the ulnar supplies the entire dorsum of the same one and a half fingers, while the radial nerve supplies the rest, including the "anatomical snuffbox" on the lateral surface of the thumb. Vibration, fine touch and proprioception information is transmitted along the myelinated dorsal column of the spinal cord, while pain, temperature, crude touch are conducted along the spinothalamic tract to the primary somatosensory cortex. The spinothalamic tract decussates at its point of origin, while the dorsal columns decussate at the lower medulla.

Causes of peripheral neuropathy can be remembered as **A-H**: **A**lcohol, **B** vitamin deficiencies (e.g. B6, B12), **C**ancer/ **C**onnective tissue diseases, **D**iabetes/**D**rugs (e.g. phenytoin), **E**verything else (e.g. vasculitides) **F**riedrich's ataxia, **G**uillain- Barré syndrome, **H**ereditary sensory-motor neuropathy (a.k.a. Charcot-Marie-Tooth syndrome).

OSCE 3 – Examination

Actor's instructions

You are tired and worried. You only reveal unprompted points about your child when asked open questions and not interrupted, but only mention key features such as vaccinations, fontanelles and rash when asked.

When asked about	You mention
Name	Hello, my name is Brenda Hopkins. My baby's 20 weeks and has been poorly the last 2 days. I took her to the GP this morning with a fever, and she gave a prescription for antibiotics and told us to give her paracetamol and plenty of fluids. Since then she's gotten worse. She's been vomiting, and she isn't taking any milk. She's been screaming the whole night, but more recently she seems to have cried herself out and is just staring. What should I do?
Fever	Her fever is 39 degrees.
Rash	She's got a rash on her leg but it blanches when I push a glass on it.
Responsiveness	She's drowsy, she responds to her name, but seems spaced out.
Fontanelles	What are they? [On answer:]: No, they're not swollen.
Neck retraction	No her neck isn't like that.
Rigors or shakes	She's not had any shakes.
Coolness of hands and feet	They are maybe a little cold, but the heating isn't on.
Vaccinations	She is up to date for her vaccinations.
Past medical health	She wasn't premature or anything, she weighed 3.3 kg at birth. She's been breastfed and hasn't

been ill apart from a few sniffles before this, which is why I'm worried.

Infected contacts   I don't know anyone with meningitis who's been near her.

Marking Scheme	
2 marks: Good - 1 mark: Adequate - 0 mark: Poor/Not done	**Mark 0 – 2**

1. Polite introduction, takes patient's name.
2. Takes presenting complaint.
3. Finds out about temperature.
4. Asks about rash.
5. Finds out about responsiveness.
6. Asks about fontanelles.
7. Asks about neck retraction.
8. Asks about coolness of peripheries.
9. Asks about rigors.
10. Asks about vaccinations.
11. Finds out about past medical health.
12. Finds out about meningitis contacts.
13. Overall impression.

Examiner's additional questions

Q: What would you recommend for her to do?
14. A: Take the baby to hospital, on suspicion of **meningitis**.

Q: If you were at the scene, talk me through the key points of your examination.
A: Explains they would:
15. ▪ take blood pressure, heart rate
16. ▪ take temperature, respiratory rate
17. ▪ assess capillary refill time (normally <2 seconds after 5 seconds pressure) and feel coolness of peripheries
18. ▪ assess consciousness (e.g. AVPU scale)
19. ▪ look for infectious focus: inflamed throat, tympanic membranes, neurological exam including testing for reaction, check all over body for rash and record

Brudzinski's and Kernig's signs, abdominal exam, respiratory exam, test pupil size and extent if it blanches, its speed of development and if it is petechial or purpuric

Q: On a home visit, what treatment would you give for bacterial meningitis?

20. **A:** Give intramuscular benzylpenicillin at the scene while awaiting ambulance (IV/IM cefotaxime in hospital). ☐

TOTAL SCORE **/ 40**

Further Information

Infants with meningitis or septicaemia will not necessarily demonstrate the classic signs. Only 10-15% of infants less than 3 months of age develop neck stiffness and 15% develop a bulging fontanelle (Rothrock and Green 2003).

AVPU scale (quick consciousness assessment tool for infants)

A	Alert	
V	Responds to Voice	
P	Responds to Pain	**P** or **U** scores correspond to a Glasgow
U	Unresponsive	Coma Scale of 8 or less.

In children under 24 months of age, **persistent fever, loss of appetite**, apparent **abdominal pain, vomiting, high-pitched cry, restlessness** and **irritability** which develops into **lethargy** suggest serious illness so their **carers provide vital history**.

Bacterial meningitis can occur without septicaemia and still be fatal; likewise, meningococcus can kill by septicaemia in the absence of meningitis. Hence meningitis should be considered, **even in the absence of non-blanching rash**.

Glasgow Coma Scale

Eyes   **4:** Open spontaneously.   **3:** Open to speech
         2: Open to pain   **1:** Do not open

Speech **5:** Normal, oriented speech   **4:** Confused but understandable
                                          speech
          3: Nonsensical speech   **2:** Vocal noises
          1: No speech

Motor **6:** Can obey a motor command   **5:** Localizes pain
         4: Non-localized withdrawal   **3:** Limb flexor response to pain
         response to pain   (decorticate)
         2: Limb extensor response to   **1:** No movement at all.
         pain (decerebrate)

UK Vaccination Timeline (NHS 2009)	
When immunised	**Diseases vaccinated against**
2 months old	Diphtheria, tetanus, pertussis (whooping cough), polio and *Haemophilus influenzae* type b (Hib)
3 months old	Diphtheria, tetanus, pertussis, polio and *Haemophilus influenzae* type b (Hib), Meningitis C
4 months old	Diphtheria, tetanus, pertussis, polio and *Haemophilus influenzae* type b (Hib), Meningitis C, Pneumococcus
Around 12 months	*Haemophilus influenza* type b (Hib), Meningitis C
Around 13 months old	Measles, mumps and rubella, Pneumococcus
3 years and 4 months or soon after	Diphtheria, tetanus, pertussis and polio, Measles, mumps and rubella
Girls aged 12 to13 years	Cervical cancer caused by human papillomavirus types 16 and 18.
13 to 18 years old	Diphtheria, tetanus, polio

OSCE 4 – History

Actor's instructions
You are tired and in pain; your history is based on the speech below. You reveal unprompted information about yourself when asked open questions and not interrupted.

When asked about	You mention
Name	Ethel Winehouse
Presenting complaint	This morning, when I woke up I had a crashing headache. I got up out of bed to close the curtains and I fell down. You see I had this awful headache, and I get these horrible burning pains in my shoulders and hips, and I tripped over my bedside table, I hadn't seen it. I'd gone blind in my right eye. Don't worry, I was fine, but it did me a mischief getting up again. I've been feeling feverish too. I knew I needed to come to hospital. I called my GP just in case and he agreed.
Site of pain	It's on the right hand side, a burning sort of pain.
Movement	It don't seem to move anywhere
Alleviating factors	Nothing they've given me helps. Aspirin doesn't touch it, neither does paracetamol.
What makes it worse	It hurts something awful when I try to comb my hair on that side.
Pain while eating	This pain on the right side of my jaw comes on whenever I'm eating. It dims down when I stop chewing for a minute, but comes back when I try to finish my meal.
Severity	I'd say it was 9 out of 10, it's awful, but what really worried me is going blind in my right eye.
Duration of symptoms	This headache has been going on for about 2 weeks I'd say. The eye problem only started this

morning though. I've been having the shoulder problem for maybe a month. But I've had arthritis in both my knees for years.

Weight loss I've been losing weight as well over the last month or so, I haven't been feeling well at all, it's not helping with my sleep neither.

Past medical history I've been quite well before this. I had my tonsils out when I was small, and I've got arthritis in both knees.

Drugs As I said, aspirin and paracetamol don't work. I'm not taking anything else.

Marking Scheme	
2 marks: Good - 1 mark: Adequate - 0 mark: Poor/Not done	**Mark 0 – 2**

1. Polite introduction, takes patient's name.
2. Takes presenting complaint: headache, sudden unilateral loss of sight, fever.

Finds out about pain:
3.   ▪ Site
4.   ▪ Onset
5.   ▪ Character
6.   ▪ Radiation
7.   ▪ Alleviating factors
8.   ▪ Timing (worse in morning)
9.   ▪ Exacerbating factors
10.   ▪ Severity
11. Finds out about claudication pain.
12. Asks about past medical history
13. Asks about drug history
14. Thanks the patient. Overall impression.

Examiner's additional questions (near the end)	
Q: What is your diagnosis? 15. A: Giant cell arteritis (a.k.a. temporal arteritis) with polymyalgia rheumatica.	☐
Q: What is the treatment required? 16. A: Urgent prednisolone and bisphosphonates would be needed to save her sight and treat her joint pain.	☐
Q: What investigations would you recommend? 17. A: Temporal artery biopsy, ESR, alkaline phosphatise	☐

TOTAL SCORE	/ 34

Further information

When taking a history of pain, it is important to know its **SOCRA-TES: S**ite, **O**nset, **C**haracter, **RA**diation, **T**iming, **E**xacerbating factors and **S**everity.

Giant cell arteritis is a large-vessel vaculitis affecting the 50+ age group. It is associated with **polymyalgia rheumatica**, also stemming from vasculitis, causing sudden pain in the proximal joints. Pain is worse in the morning and lasts hours, felt over the temporal and/or occipital arteries, which are swollen, tortuous, pulseless and hardened. **Jaw claudication** is painful muscle ischaemia due to involvement of the maxillary branch of the external carotid artery. Sudden, painless, unilateral loss of eyesight (**amaurosis fugax**) usually results from inflammation of the posterior ciliary artery. ESR is normally elevated, reaching 60-100 mm/hour, with **temporal artery biopsy** producing definitive diagnosis. With a suggestive clinical picture and amaurosis fugax, high-dose prednisolone is started before biopsy, with bisphosphonates to prevent bone thinning.

Corticosteroids are the major cause of long-term morbidity in giant cell arteritis (iatrogenic Cushing's disease). Long-term treatment is needed as the risk of blindness persists; specialist advice is required when considering cessation, with gradual reduction to avoid iatrogenic Addison's syndrome (underactive adrenal glands). ~25% of patients still require treatment after 3 years.

OSCE 5 – History

Actor's instructions
You are tired and uncomfortable; you reveal unprompted symptoms when asked open questions and not interrupted.

When asked about	You mention
Name	Hello, I'm Beth Garner.
Symptoms	Just the last week or so, I've been feeling tired all the time. It's come on all of a sudden. I start the day tired, and it carries on. Normally I'm running about doing everything, but I've had to really cut down. My sister says it could be depression, but it's more than just tiredness. I'm getting a bit of pain and I think my eyesight's going a bit, all blurry in my left, plus I'm getting a sort of tingling in my legs and they're weak.
Any pain?	I get a sharp pain just in my left eye, more when I look around, nothing that bad. Again it's just been the last week. The tingling in my legs isn't a pain as such, sometimes it's more like numbness.
Does it move Anywhere?	No.
What makes pain worse	The pain in my left eye, and the blurriness, seems to get worse when I have a shower and when I move it.
What makes pain better	Nothing really makes it better; it comes and goes on its own.
How long it lasts for	It lasts at its worst about 15 minutes in bursts over a few days.
Previous episodes	I had something similar about eight months ago. My GP couldn't do anything about it, he said come back if it happens again, then it lasted about a month and went on its own.

138

Past medical history	I've been healthy most of my life. I had pneumonia when I was 11, that's the only time I've been to hospital, I've never had any operations
Drug history	I'm not on any medication.
Family history	Well, I've got 2 grandparents still alive, one died of a stroke aged 82, the other had a heart attack aged 75. My parents are in good health, so is my sister.
Effect on your life	I'm a social worker and I've been off sick for the last 3 days. Work's been hectic, but not anything worse than usual. Yesterday, I had to call my sister up to plck my daughter from school, because I was just too tired, you know? And I don't like doing that, she's got her own responsibilities. Even doing the shopping, getting about is much more tiring than it should be. I wouldn't say I was depressed, maybe a bit stressed, but everyone's stressed aren't they?

Marking Scheme

2 marks: Good - 1 mark: Adequate - 0 mark: Poor/Not done	Mark 0 – 2
1. Polite introduction, verifies identity.	☐
2. Takes presenting complaint (tiredness, blurred vision, tingling, weakness, pain)	☐
3. Finds site of pain.	☐
4. Finds when pain started.	☐
5. Finds character of pain.	☐
6. Asks about pain radiating.	☐
7. Asks what makes pain better.	☐
8. Asks what makes pain worse.	☐
9. Asks about timing of pain.	☐
10. Asks about pain severity.	☐
11. Asks about previous episodes.	☐
12. Asks about past medical history	☐
13. Asks about family history.	☐

14. Asks about medication.	☐
15. Asks about effects on her life.	☐
16. Thanks the patient. Overall impression.	☐

Examiner's additional questions (near the end)

Q: What is the diagnosis?
17. **A:** Suspected multiple sclerosis. ☐

TOTAL SCORE / 34

Further information

Multiple sclerosis causes **plaques** of **demyelination** in the **CNS**, often described as "disseminated in time and space" (i.e. occurring in different brain regions at different times). Clinical features include eye pain and diplopia (optic neuritis), trigeminal neuralgia, nystagmus, depression, fatigue, tingling, UMN signs, cerebellar signs, urinary urgency and frequency incontinence, constipation and erectile dysfunction. **Uhthoff's sign**, described in the history, occurs when motor and visual symptoms worsen with increased temperature (due to further slowing of conduction). **L'Hermitte's sign** occurs when neck flexion causes tingling in the arms and legs and is also seen in cervical spondylosis and vitamin B12 deficiency. Colour vision (particularly reds) is often impaired with optic neuritis, this can be tested with an Ishihara chart.

Symptoms are typically **relapsing and remitting** but this can develop into a **secondary progressive** form with gradual accumulation of symptoms. ~20% of cases follow a **primary progressive** pattern, with gradual worsening from the start, while <10% follow a **fulminant** path, with no intervening remissions. Relapse episodes can be shortened by high-dose IV corticosteroids. Beta interferon therapy may reduce the frequency of recurrences. Urine retention (due to sphincter spasticity) can lead to kidney damage and should be treated with intermittent self-catheterisation, while urgency (exaggerated bladder reflexes) can be treated by oxybutynin. Motor spasticity is treated with muscle relaxants such as dantrolene. Fluoxetine is recommended if depression develops as it has minimal anticholinergic effects (such as urinary retention, constipation, dry mouth and confusion). With further progression, care assistance, support groups, physiotherapy, home and workplace adaptations are beneficial. Poor prognostic factors include a short interval between 1st and 2nd episodes, older age at onset and being male.

OSCE 6 – History

Actor's instructions
You are in pain and irritable; you don't mention your bladder and sexual problems unless specifically asked, but are more likely to volunteer other unprompted symptoms when asked open questions and not interrupted.

When asked about	You mention
Name	Hello I'm Clement Battersby.
Symptoms	Well just yesterday, I was doing some gardening, and I had to lift this metal table. I wasn't concentrating cos I was listening to the radio. Obviously, you're meant to bend at your knees, especially with my back problems, but I didn't and I did my back in. I almost screamed it was that bad, it still canes now.
Type of pain	I'd say it's just kind of short and stabbing, fizzing sort of pain.
The pain moving anywhere	It goes down both my legs.
Drugs taken to alleviate the pain	I've taken some codeine at home, that's taken some of the edge off it.
Timing of pain	Again, it got worse last night, I've had problems before, taking codeine's maybe taken a little edge off it but not much.
If anything makes the pain worse	Lifting, I'd imagine, something I've not been stupid enough to try since yesterday.
Severity out of 10	I'd say, really this is as bad as it's ever been, maybe an 8 out of 10.
Back problem history	My back? I'm in here all the time for my back. I'd say it's been giving me problems on and off for about 10 years. I'm a builder and I've lost work

days sometimes, spasms.

Most of the time I can get through. I don't like coming to the doctor's normally I took a day off work to come because the lady at reception said that's the only slot available.

Normally I just take paracetamol or aspirin or codeine and I'm okay, but today it's worse than that. I've never had any operations for it, or injections.

Leg weakness	I'd say maybe I'm not hundred percent at the moment. I can walk about fine, but if you were to ask me to run, that would probably be a problem.
Changes in bowel function	No, I haven't had any problems with my bowels.
Changes in bladder function	Maybe a little, I've been having to go more often recently.
Changes in sexual function	Well, last night, I was with my girlfriend, and there was a problem like with my groin, it could get hard but it felt a little numb; so did my kind of arse area, but no one touched it.
Past medical history	I'm quite healthy normally, never been to hospital, never had anything serious.
Family history	My dad had a few back problems, so did my mum.
Medication	I've taken some codeine for it, but I'm not on anything else.

Marking Scheme	
2 marks: Good - 1 mark: Adequate - 0 mark: Poor/Not done	**Mark 0 – 2**

1.	Polite introduction, verifies identity.	□
	Finds about pain:	
2.	▪ Site	□
3.	▪ Onset	□
4.	▪ Character	□
5.	▪ Radiation	□
6.	▪ Alleviating factors	□
7.	▪ Timing	□
8.	▪ Exacerbating factors	□
9.	▪ Severity	□
10.	Asks about changes in bowel function.	
11.	Asks about changes in bladder function: frequency, incontinence, feeling of fullness.	□
12.	Asks about sexual function: sensation, erection, ejaculation.	□
13.	Asks about leg weakness.	
14.	Finds out about past back problems and treatment.	
15.	Asks out about past medical history.	
16.	Asks about family history.	
17.	Finds out about medication.	
18.	Thanks the patient. Overall impression.	□

Examiner's additional questions (near the end)	

	Q: What is your diagnosis?	
19.	**A:** Suspected cauda equina syndrome.	□
	Q: What would you look for on examination?	
20.	**A:** Would test perineal sensation, anal tone, leg reflexes and strength.	□
	Q: What is the treatment?	
21.	**A:** Treatment is surgical urgent decompression by laminectomy.	□

TOTAL SCORE	/ 42

Further information
Cauda equina syndrome results when nerve roots are compressed as they emerge from the bottom of the spinal cord below L1. Causes include disc herniation, tumours, surgery, abscesses and haematomas. Lower back pain is a very common problem, so it is important to be wary of **red flags**, which include **leg weakness**, **severe back pain** with **unilateral or bilateral sciatica**, **sensory disturbance** in the **buttock, perineal** or **genital** areas, **sexual dysfunction**, **bladder** or **bowel dysfunction** and **gait disturbances** (Anthony 2003).

The commonest levels affected are **L4/L5** and **L5/S1** (Akbar and Mahar 2004). Shapiro (2000) found that 70% of people with cauda equina syndrome presented with a history of chronic back pain with gradual worsening over weeks and months. MRI is the gold standard for cauda equina imaging, though CT with myelography is also of use. Shapiro (2000) found that early decompressive surgery, within 48 hours, improved the chances of complete recovery.

OSCE 7 – Examination

Marking Scheme	
2 marks: Good - 1 mark: Adequate - 0 mark: Poor/Not done	**Mark 0 – 2**
1. Polite introduction.	☐
2. Asks if they wear contact lenses or glasses, whereupon examiner produces a pair of glasses.	☐
3. Student asks if they are long or short-sighted/ notes if glasses are biconvex (for long-sightedness) or biconcave (for short-sightedness).	☐
4. Explains acuity testing.	☐
5. Tests visual acuity of the examiner, without glasses, at the right distance (e.g. 6 metres) for one eye.	
6. Repeats acuity testing on the other eye.	☐
7. Gives correct acuity scores, e.g. 6/6. The line at which they get more than 50% of letters correct is their score, if they get 2 letters on that line wrong, then their score would be 6/6 -2, if they got all the letters on that row correct plus 2 from the row below, their score would be 6/6+2.	☐
8. If their vision is less than 6/6, explains they would repeat using a pinhole to correct for refractive error.	☐
9. Dims the lights. Mentions use of tropicamide eye drops.	☐
10. Explains fundoscopy: warns about bright light, asks them to fixate upon a distant point, and says they are allowed to blink.	
11. Candidate removes their own glasses, if they have any, turns on fundoscope, approaching model from eye-level ~1m away.	☐
12. Uses right eye to look at model's right eye, avoids touching model's eye with fundoscope.	☐
13. Notes presence or absence of red reflex.	☐
14. Adjusts fundoscope lens, dependent on their own long/ short-sightedness and area of eye viewed. Starting at +20 enables viewing of cornea and lens. Moving towards 0 enables deeper eye structures like the fundus to be viewed.	
15. Comments correctly on optic disc, macula and vessels and retinal veins seen on slide in model eye.	☐
16. Thanks the patient, Overall impression.	☐

Examiner's additional questions (near the end)

17. **Q: What would you expect to see in glaucoma?**
    A: Describes glaucoma briefly e.g. pale disc showing optic atrophy, cupped optic disc, cloudy cornea, red eye. ☐

18. **Q: What would you expect to see with cataract?**
    A: Describes cataract briefly e.g. loss of red reflex, or an opacity silhouetted against it. ☐

19. **Q: What would you expect to see with diabetic retinopathy?**
    A: Describes diabetic retinopathy briefly e.g. background (dots and blots), pre-proliferative (cotton wool spots, venous beading), proliferative (new vessels, vitreous haemorrhage), advanced (retinal detachment, fibrosis), maculopathy (hard exudates and haemorrhages in the macular area), treated (grid pattern of laser photocoagulation scars). ☐

20. **Q: What would you expect to see with hypertensive retinopathy?**
    A: Describes hypertensive retinopathy briefly e.g. silver wiring (arteriosclerosis) progressing to arteriovenous nipping, haemorrhages, soft and hard exudates, with advanced cases causing papilloedema. ☐

TOTAL SCORE **/ 40**

Further information

The shrinking letters on the acuity chart represent sizes readable from maximum set distances by a person with normal eyesight. The largest letters forming the top line are normally legible 60m away. The measure **6/60** means that the person can only resolve from **6m** away letters that should normally be readable from **60m**. 6/5 eyesight is better than average, meaning the person can read letters from 6m away that are normally only readable from 5m. Dimming the lights or use of tropicamide (anticholinergic) eye drops causes pupils to dilate, giving a better view of the retina. Placing a hand on the patient's forehead enables better gauging of proximity, to avoid poking the patient in the eye. The **red reflex** is caused by light reflected off the retina. Absence of the red reflex indicates opacity anterior to the fundus, which can be caused by cataract, retinoblastoma, corneal scarring or vitreous haemorrhage.

The optic nerve reaches the retina at the optic disc which can be located by tracing the retinal veins to their central meeting point. **Papilloedema** is swelling of the optic disc with the loss of its slight cupping and is caused by raised intracranial pressure. Exaggerated cupping is caused by the raised intra-ocular pressure of **acute glaucoma**.

Proliferative diabetic retinopathy involves the formation of new vessels, which can cause blindness by fibrosis and retinal detachment. Diabetic patients with background changes require annual screening, while more advanced retinopathy requires referral to an ophthalmologist, urgently with proliferative or advanced changes. The UKPDS (1998) and DCCT (1993) cohort trials found that tight glucose control could prevent diabetic retinopathy in type 1 and type 2 diabetes. Proliferative diabetic retinopathy is treated with laser photocoagulation and this shows on fundoscopy as grids of light yellow circles. The causes of **cataracts** include old age, diabetes, congenital rubella and trauma.

AIDS-defining **CMV retinitis** can lead to rapid blindness, causing characteristic perivascular haemorrhages and soft exudates, typically presenting with CD4 count <100/mm^3. This requires antiretroviral therapy (starting at the right time prevents AIDS complications) and foscarnet or ganciclovir to treat CMV, which can sometimes be injected into the vitreous humour. **Central retinal artery occlusion** causes oedema, with a pale white fundus and thin retinal arteries. Examination of the entire retina is required to diagnose **retinitis pigmentosa**, characterised by peripheral black dots. Retinitis pigmentosa is the commonest form of retinal degeneration, with consequent loss of night vision and peripheral sight.

OSCE 8 – History

Actor instructions
The pain around your mouth makes you speak with as little movement as possible. In the course of speaking, you wince from one or two brief jolts of pain. You are more likely to reveal symptoms unprompted when asked open questions and not interrupted.

When asked about	You mention
Name	Hello. I'm Lena Radebe.
Symptoms	I've got this awful pain right here (points without touching to left of mouth), it's really sharp, sort of electric shock type of pain. Ow. That's it right there. I've had it for about a week and it's becoming difficult to concentrate at work. I've never had anything like it before.
If it moves anywhere	No, it just stays in that kind of area.
If anything helps with the pain	I tried taking aspirin but it didn't work at all.
Timing	It just comes on for a few seconds each time during the day. It tends to be worse when I touch it, or move that part of my face. Like in the morning, I might forget and slap cold water on it first thing and then it really kicks. Brushing my teeth in the morning and night it's quite bad, and mealtimes, any contact in that sort of area makes it come on.
Severity out of 10	When it comes on, just for a few seconds, it's almost like labour pain, 7 out of 10.
Past medical history	I'm quite healthy otherwise. A few years ago I was getting chest pain, but my GP told me to take a few days off work and it was fine. I had asthma when I was a kid, but nothing serious at all.
Family history	I've not heard of anyone in my family having any-

thing like this. My parents are still alive and healthy, so is my older brother.

Medication   Like I say, I took some aspirin, but nothing else and it didn't work anyway.

How it is affecting your life   I've taken today off work, because it's stressing me out. I work as a teacher in a secondary school and I didn't feel I had the strength to face a class of 30 today.

Marking Scheme	
2 marks: Good - 1 mark: Adequate - 0 mark: Poor/Not done	**Mark 0 – 2**
1. Polite introduction; takes patient's name.	☐
2. Finds out about presenting complaint.	
Finds out about pain:	
3. ▪ Site	☐
4. ▪ Onset	
5. ▪ Character	
6. ▪ Radiation	
7. ▪ Alleviating factors	
8. ▪ Time pattern	
9. ▪ Exacerbating factors	
10. ▪ Severity	
11. Asks about past medical history.	
12. Asks about medication.	
13. Asks about family history.	
14. Asks about social effects.	
15. Thanks the patient. Overall impression.	☐
Examiner's additional questions (near the end)	
Q: What is your diagnosis?	
16. **A:** Trigeminal neuralgia.	☐

Q: What would you look for on examination?
17. **A:** Test motor and sensory function of trigeminal nerve. ☐
Trigeminal neuralgia tends not to affect these functions, but other causes of trigeminal pain can.

Q: What is the treatment?
18. **A:** Carbamazepine is first-choice. ☐

TOTAL SCORE / 36

Further Information

Trigeminal neuralgia tends to affect older people, with an incidence of ~20 per 100 000 people per year in the over-60's and is **mostly idiopathic**, though it can be caused by multiple sclerosis, with other causes of pain in this distribution including herpes zoster, syringobulbia, internal carotid artery aneurysm and cavernous sinus thrombosis. The pain is typically **unilateral**, stabbing (**lasting seconds**) and in the maxillary or mandibular dermatome. It can cause a wincing, known as **tic douloureux**, but is typically **absent at night**. It can be exacerbated by skin contact, eating, speaking and brushing the teeth. Motor and sensory functions tend to remain intact in true trigeminal neuralgia, though these may be impaired by other causes of trigeminal pain.

First-line treatment includes the anti-epileptic carbamazepine. Neuropathic pain stems from hyperexcitable nerves as opposed to tissue damage, and may be related to descending facilitatory pain signals; opiates have little efficacy. If carbamazepine doesn't work, unlicensed treatments include lamotrigine, gabapentin and clonazepam. Some refractory cases are deemed suitable for surgical interventions such as thermocoagulation, alcohol injection and neurovascular decompression. It tends to follow a relapsing course, with remissions lasting months or years.

OSCE 9 – History

Actor instructions

You have pain and weakness in your left hand. You reveal more un-prompted symptoms when asked open questions and not interrupted.

When asked about	You mention
Name	Hello, my name is Nazma Hossain.
Your problem	I've got this tingling pain in my left hand, especially the middle finger. It's difficult to carry the shopping and to type on the computer. It's been going on for 2 or 3 weeks and isn't going away on its own.
Where specifically	My middle finger on the left side.
If the pain moves	No it just seems to stay in my hand
If anything makes it better	Nothing seems to make it better, I've taken some aspirin, that's it. Maybe at night, if I give my wrist a shake, or hand it off the edge of the bed I can get back to sleep.
Timing	I wouldn't say it's constant. It's worse at night.
What worsens it	It seems to get worse when I'm typing.
Severity out of 10	I'd say it was 6 out of 10.
Left/ right handed?	I'm left handed.
Past medical history	I'd say I'm quite healthy, never had an operation, never been to hospital.
Conditions	I don't have diabetes, arthritis or hypothyroidism.
Medication	I'm on the oral contraceptive pill, and tried aspirin.
Job	I work at a meat-packing plant, chopping carcasses all day.

Marking Scheme

2 marks: Good - 1 mark: Adequate - 0 mark: Poor/Not done	Mark 0 – 2
1. Polite introduction; takes patient's name.	☐
2. Finds out about presenting complaint.	☐
Finds out about pain:	
3. ▪ Site	☐
4. ▪ Onset	☐
5. ▪ Character	☐
6. ▪ Radiation	☐
7. ▪ Alleviating factors	☐
8. ▪ Time pattern	☐
9. ▪ Exacerbating factors	☐
10. ▪ Severity	☐
11. Asks about past medical history.	☐
12. Asks about predisposing conditions e.g. diabetes, arthritis hypothyroidism.	☐
13. Finds if they are left or right handed.	☐
14. Asks about medication.	☐
15. Asks about job.	☐
16. Thanks the patient. Overall impression.	☐

Examiner's additional questions (near the end)

Q: What is your diagnosis?
17. **A:** Carpal tunnel syndrome. ☐

Q: What would you look for on examination?
18. **A:** On examination: explains Tinel's and Phalen's signs may Be present, explains pen-touching test for weakness of the abductor pollicis brevis. ☐

Q: What is the treatment?
19. **A:** Splinting, steroid injections, surgical decompression of carpal tunnel. ☐

TOTAL SCORE | / 38

Further information
Phalen's test is holding the wrist in flexion for 60 seconds, which can provoke tingling pain symptoms in the median nerve region. Tinel's test is
tapping over the flexor retinaculum where the median nerve passes,
which again can provoke tingling symptoms.

Tinel's test may be remembered by it involving **t**apping, while
Phalen's involves **fl**exion.

However, neither Phalen's nor Tinel's is particularly reliable, and diagnosis of carpal tunnel syndrome is based mainly on history. The **abductor
pollicis brevis** muscle may be weak and is tested by the **pen-touching
test**, whereby the hand is placed palm up on a flat surface and the patient
is asked to touch a pen by bringing their thumb up vertically.

All the intrinsic muscles of the hand are supplied by the ulnar
nerve except the **LOAF** muscles: 2 lateral **L**umbricals, **O**pponens
pollicis, **A**bductor pollicis brevis and **F**lexor pollicis brevis (all supplied by the median nerve).

Median nerve palsy can cause an **ape hand deformity** (loss of thumb
opposition), with sensation affected over the palmar surface of the thumb,
index and middle fingers. **Ulnar palsy** causes **clawing** of the ring and
little finger- flexion at the interphalangeal joints and extension at the metacarpophalangeal joints, with sensation affected over the palmar and dorsal surfaces of the little finger. This is more pronounced with lesion at the
wrist because flexor digitorum profundus function remains, enabling flexion at the interphalangeal joints.

OSCE 10 – Written station: investigations

1 – F

In myasthenia gravis, autoantibodies are directed against post-synaptic acetylcholine receptors. Edrophonium is a short-acting acetylcholinesterase inhibitor that temporarily increases the availability of acetylcholine at the neuromuscular junction, causing a transient improvement in motor function. Resuscitation facilities are required for this test because acetylcholine can cause cardiac arrest. Myasthenia gravis causes weakness worsened by activity, particularly affecting proximal muscles found at the orbits, throat, face (producing "myasthenic snarl" on attempted smile) and shoulder girdle.

Clinical tests include asking the patient to blink repeatedly for a minute, maintain prolonged upward gaze, or count aloud to 50, all of which demonstrate progressive weakening; applying an ice cube to the eye for 2 minutes can reduce ptosis by more than 2mm in someone with myasthenia gravis. Other investigations include serology, nerve conduction studies, thymus CT scan (~10% of cases associated with thymomas) and single nerve fiber electromyography (declining response on repeated stimulation).

Myasthenia gravis is associated with other autoimmune diseases like pernicious anaemia, systemic lupus erythematosus and Hashimoto's thyroiditis. Treatment includes long-acting acetylcholinesterase inhibitors (e.g. pyridostigmine), thymectomy, prednisolone and azothioprine immunosuppression and plasmapheresis.

2 – E

EMG tongue fibrillations are spontaneous contractions of hyperexcitable individual muscle fibers following denervation and pathognomic of **motor neurone disease**.

3 – G

On the **EMG** speakers, this waxing and waning frequency pattern can be likened to a stopping and starting motorcycle engine and is characteristic of **myotonia**. Percussion myotonia is elicited by tapping the thenar eminence, which causes contraction then gradual relaxation of the abductor pollicis brevis.

4 – A

3Hz spike and wave EEG activity is characteristic of **absence seizures** (AKA petit mal). These are a form of generalized seizure, hence the wide-spread signal disturbance. Valproate is a first-line treatment for adult absence seizures, with other options including lamotrigine and ethosuximide (NICE October 2004).

5 – J

Tonic seizures are characterized by generalized **EEG activity** at **10Hz** or faster. First-line treatments include valproate and lamotrigine (NICE 2004).

6 – I

Tonic clonic seizures (AKA grand mal) are characterized by generalized **EEG activity** at **10Hz** followed by **slower signals** or **mixed slow waves** and **spikes**. Clinical features after a tonic clonic seizure include a bitten tongue, incontinence, bilateral upward plantar reflexes, exaggerated reflexes and weakness (Todd's paresis). First-line treatments include lamotrigine, topiramate valproate and carbamazepine (NICE 2004).

7 – H

The nerve conduction study would ascertain the location of nerve injury. The intact peripheral nerve suggests proximal damage such as **nerve root avulsion**. This would be less likely to regenerate than a peripheral nerve injury.

8 – D

Mononeuritis multiplex is the most likely diagnosis when conduction is reduced at several sites that are not typically subject to nerve compression. Nerves at widespread locations are involved as opposed to the glove and stocking distribution affecting adjacent nerves in peripheral neuropathy. Mononeuritis multiplex is caused by diabetes, HIV, sarcoidosis, leprosy and Guillain-Barré syndrome.

9 – C

Transient increases in muscle response can be as high as 200% on repeated nerve stimulation in **Lambert-Eaton syndrome.** Thus, on examination, strength improves on repetitive movements. This **paraneoplastic syndrome (**associated with small cell lung cancer) has similar symptoms to myasthenia gravis. Rather than being directed against post-synaptic receptors, antibodies are directed against the **presynaptic membrane**, reflexes tend to be impaired, there is only a slight response to edrophonium and peripheral muscles are affected before proximal. As it can develop years before lung cancer, regular chest x rays are required. Symptoms may be alleviated by 3, 4-diaminopyridine.

10 – B

Carpal tunnel syndrome is caused by **median nerve compression** under the flexor retinaculum and is associated with prolonged typing, pregnancy, diabetes, hypothyroidism and arthritis. The median nerve distribution is affected- the index, middle finger and thumb, with aching pain worst at night. Weakness and wasting of the thenar eminence may also occur. Tinel's test involves repeated tapping over the flexor retinaculum and asking if it causes tingling in the fingers. Phalen's test involves holding the hands in a reverse prayer position (both wrists flexed against each other) for 1 minute and asking if it causes pain. Treatments include physiotherapy, decompression, splinting and hydrocortisone injection.

OSCE 11 – Written station: Neuro-imaging

1 – G

Demyelination in **multiple sclerosis** is detected by MRI T2 imaging (the first-line modality for MS), and can be found in the spinal cord, around ventricles, brainstem, optic nerve, cerebellum and corpus callosum, with active plaques enhanced by with gadolinium. The **sunray sign** is key, with lesions resembling straight beams emerging from the callosal margin to the cortex on **sagittal MRI** T2-weighted views. MRIs taken with the progression of MS show <u>lesions disseminated in time and space</u> (i.e. multiple clinical events affecting multiple regions of the CNS). Plaques can be confluent and may appear as a single large lesion on MRI, whereupon the differential of a space occupying lesion should be considered, particularly as the symptoms caused by CNS lymphoma may also regress with corticosteroid therapy. This type of presentation could necessitate biopsy. Visual **evoked potentials** are measured by monitoring visual, cortex signals by EEG while the patient receives visual stimulation. Similar delays can be detected at the auditory or somatosensory cortex on auditory or tactile stimulation. Optic nerve demyelination causes the signal to be delayed but with amplitude preserved.

2 – D

Extradural haematomas accumulate between the dura and bone. As they tend to be **arterial** and higher-pressure bleeds than subdural haemorrhages, they displace the brain more, causing a rounded shape on **CT** described as **biconvex** or **lenticular**. They may cross the midline but tend not to cross skull suture lines.

3 – C

Brain affected by **CVA** has **reduced density** on **CT**. **MRI** shows **infarcted brain areas** as **hypointense on T1** and **hyperintense on T2** (due to oedema). MRI is more sensitive to early CVA than CT. The wedge shape reflects the region supplied by the blocked vessel. Haemorrhagic infarction on CT causes spots of high density (fresh blood) within areas of low density (infarcted brain).

4 – F

This is characteristic of **meningioma**, a benign tumour of the dura mater. **CT** is often preferred for their detection, as they display **high density** and are **enhancing**.

5 – A

This **ring-enhancing lesion** is due to a thickened **abscess** wall. **MRI T2 highlights oedema**, hence is better at detecting abscesses. They can extend from infected bone and sinuses or be embolized from infectious loci, such as diseased heart valves or decayed teeth. There may be extradural accumulation of pus and when multiple lesions are present, differential diagnosis encompasses tuberculomas, sarcoidosis and metastases.

6 – H

CT is more sensitive than MRI to these areas of **calcification** caused by quiescent **neurocysticercosis** infection.

7 – E

Gliomas are tumours of glial support cells in the CNS. On **CT**, they display **low density**, mass effect (e.g. shrunken ventricles, herniation, midline shift, compression of sulci) and **irregular enhancement** with more **aggressive varieties** disrupting the blood-brain barrier.

8 – I

Sarcoidosis is a chronic inflammatory condition which gives rise to **non-caseating granuloma** formation mostly at the lungs, though any part of the body can be affected, causing restrictive lung disease and fibrosis, fatigue, weight loss, blurred vision, lymphadenopathy, aseptic meningitis and facial nerve palsy. Prevalence is raised amongst Afro-Caribbean people and it is associated with coeliac disease (inflammatory bowel reaction to glutens). Treatment is with corticosteroids and other immunosuppressants. Most experience a spontaneous remission, though 20% require steroids and 20% have persistent severe symptoms despite therapy.

9 – J

Crescent-shaped or **concave convex** haematomas are characteristic of **subdural haemorrhage**. These tend to be venous in nature, with low flow rates and accumulation over weeks. They tend not to cross the midline, but may cross skull suture lines. There may be features of mass effect like herniation, ventricular collapse, midline shift and compressed sulci. **Fresh blood** appears **hyperdense** on **CT**, though after **2 or more weeks** the haemoglobin breaks down and subdural bleeds appear **iso- or hypo-dense**.

10 – B

Cerebral metastases tend to demonstrate strong **enhancement**, with **surrounding oedema** and can be multiple.

Further information

When analyzing a scan, the patient's name, the date, type of scan (plus T1 or T2 weighting with MRI) and axis (all **CT brain images are in the axial axis**, i.e. a horizontal slice) should be noted first. Axial images in CT or MRI are viewed as if looking up from the patient's toes, thus features on the left of the image are on the right of the patient's brain. CT uses x-ray radiation which make **low-density mediums** appear **dark** (CSF, blood after 2 weeks and air), while **high- density mediums** appear **light** (fresh blood, brain calcification and bone). **Calcification** can be normal at the basal ganglia, pineal gland, falx cerebri and choroid plexus but can also be caused by **neurocysticercosis, CMV encephalitis, tuberculosis, tumours** and **gliosis** following injury. **Iodine** is used as a **CT contrast agent** to highlight areas of blood-brain barrier compromise and areas of increased vascularity.

MRI uses pulses of powerful magnetic fields to align hydrogen ions, which emit detectable radiofrequency signals when the field is removed, and are analyzed by T1 and T2 weighting. Tissue on MRI is described by the intensity of signal it emits, while on CT it is described by density and attenuation- the extent to which it blocks x-rays. MRI T1 weighting gives high acuity images (CT may miss lesions smaller than 1 cm in diameter), showing flowing **blood** as **low intensity** (black) and **fat** as **high intensity** (white).

MRI uses gadolinium-labelled DTPA as a contrast agent and doesn't involve harmful radiation, but can't be used on people with metal in their bodies. MRI provides greater anatomical detail than CT, producing images in any plane, but is slower and more expensive. CT is preferred for acute head injury and bone imaging and is often needed to discount space occupying lesions prior to lumbar puncture, thus preventing death by brainstem coning. MRI is best for soft tissue imaging and detecting white matter disease, oedema (on T2), spinal cord pathology, abscesses, arteriovenous malformations, posterior fossa tumours (using gadolinium-labelled DTPA) and acute CVA's not detected on CT.

OSCE 12 – Explaining Alzheimer's disease

Actor instructions
You are worried for your mother. You only say what you know so far if asked. If the doctor tells you the results of tests, you ask him to explain them.

When asked about	You mention
Name	Good morning. My name is Edith Rogers.
What you know so far	My mother was diagnosed 2 weeks ago with moderate Alzheimer's disease. I knew that she was having memory problems. She is quite mobile, recognises me, my kids and the rest of the family.
Your mother's living arrangements	My mother is semi-independent at the moment. She lives in sheltered accommodation with a carer who visits every morning, makes her breakfast and clears the place up. She has friends in her building.
Family support	My brother knows about the diagnosis, but he hardly comes to see her anyway. I live a mile away with my 3 daughters, but I still do all her shopping for her. My mother has 2 sisters, both older than her. They live nearby and are quite healthy and independent and know about the diagnosis. They visit quite often. My father died 4 years ago. She was depressed for maybe a year, but seems better now.
If you have any questions	How can you be sure it's Alzheimer's? What is Alzheimer's? What else could it be? What treatment is available? How long has she got left? Does this mean I'll get Alzheimer's too? Where can I find out more?

Marking Scheme	
2 marks: Good - 1 mark: Adequate - 0 mark: Poor/Not done	**Mark 0 – 2**

1. Polite introduction; verifies the patient's identity. ☐
2. Asks what she knows so far. ☐
3. Explains symptoms: progressive memory impairment, loss of independence. ☐
4. Finds out about current living arrangements. ☐
5. Finds out about family support. ☐
6. Explains tests and why they were done- to rule out some causes of treatable impaired cognition. ☐
7. Mentions her mother may wish to choose someone with power of attorney, nominated to make financial decisions. ☐
8. Mentions her mother may need an improved care package. ☐
9. Asks for questions. ☐
10. Explains that the diagnosis of Alzheimer's is based on a memory assessment, history, examination and investigations to exclude some of the other causes.
11. Explains what Alzheimer's dementia is- e.g. the commonest form of dementia (~50% of cases), causing persisting and progressive memory problems, affecting spatial memory and recall of events. Alzheimer's initially damages brain structures responsible for memory and learning, with gradual spread to other areas and worsening function. ☐
12. Explains there is no cure currently, but there are treatments which can help some people. ☐
13. Explains there are other less common forms of dementia, e.g. multiple infarct dementia which causes a stepwise progressive dementia, frontotemporal dementia, which is also progressive and incurable. ☐
14. Explains she is being evaluated for drug therapy and further testing (e.g. CT scans) by a specialist team. Alzheimer's treatment is only suitable for some patients, potentially slowing the advance of dementia, and has side-effects. ☐
15. Explains that people can survive for years with Alzheimer's, though quality of life declines with advanced disease. ☐
16. Explains that Alzheimer's is very common in old age (~20% of those aged 80 or more have at least a mild form). Just ☐

because her mother has developed it in old age, it doesn't necessarily mean she will.

17. Explains interventions available- visiting carers, day centres, care homes for advanced disease, treatments of other illnesses which can worsen mental function. ☐

18. Offers to give her a leaflet or suggests an organisation on the internet e.g. Alzheimers.org.uk (at which point examiner hands her a leaflet). ☐

19. Overall impression. ☐

TOTAL SCORE / 38

Further information

Dementia is a **sustained reduction** in mental functioning sufficient to cause a **significant reduction in daily functioning without impairment of consciousness** (this would be acute confusional state). **Alzheimer's** causes ~50% of cases, with prevalence 5-10% above 65 years of age and ~20% above 80. Other causes include multiple infarct dementia (~25%), frontotemporal dementia, Lewy body dementia, HIV encephalopathy and Huntington's chorea. There is often a combination of causes, e.g. Alzheimer's and multiple infarct dementia; vascular risk factors are associated with increased prevalence of dementia in old age. Reversible or partially reversible causes of impaired cognition include carbon monoxide toxicity, depression, drugs, hypothyroidism, vitamin B1, B12 or folate deficiency, neurosyphilis, subdural haemorrhage, colloid cyst and normal pressure hydrocephalus. With loss of independence, people may be forced to sell their property to fund their care. According the Mental Capacity Act (2005), people with impaired competence can give a friend or relative "**enduring power of attorney**", meaning they can manage their finances, while "**lasting power of attorney**" gives influence on financial, health and welfare decisions. Furthermore, vulnerable adults without family or friends should be appointed an Independent Mental Capacity Advocate (IMCA), to help them have more say in important health-related decisions, or to represent them when there is no one else to offer support. Current Alzheimer's treatments, such as reversible acetylcholinesterase inhibitors (e.g. donezipil) and NMDA receptor antagonists (e.g. memantine), may sometimes produce slight improvements, but side-effects can be severe. Immunisation against beta amyloid plaques is a potential treatment under research (Schenk 2002).

OSCE 13 – Epilepsy advice

Actor instructions
You reveal more when asked open questions and not interrupted. You don't mention driving eligibility unless the candidate brings it up.

When asked about	You mention
Name	I'm Jennifer White
Experience so far	I have had 3 seizures and was diagnosed a week ago with epilepsy. My last fit was 2 weeks ago in an English lesson. I could tell it was going to happen, it started in my left hand, then I blacked out and woke up on the floor. It was the most embarrassing experience in my life so far. Since my first fit 3 months ago, I've stopped my driving lessons and quit an evening job at a supermarket. I'm taking the medication but it makes me feel drowsy and less sharp.
Other medication	I'm not on any other medication, I've been well my whole life, otherwise.
Drug / alcohol use	I don't drink very much. Maybe a few cans of cider at a party. Sometimes I smoke weed when I get stressed, but I don't touch anything else.
If you have any questions	I have some exams coming up, would it be okay to stop my medication to improve my concentration?

The examiner has a hidden leaflet which they hand to Ms White if the candidate mentions written information.

Marking Scheme	
2 marks: Good - 1 mark: Adequate – 0 mark: Poor/Not done	**Mark 0 – 2**

1. Polite introduction, verifies patient's name. ☐
2. Finds out about extent of current illness. ☐
3. Asks if the patient is on any other medication. ☐
4. Asks about alcohol and drug use. ☐
5. Advises her to avoid drinking and using drugs (particularly stimulants such as cocaine) due to increased seizure risk. ☐
6. Advises the patient about precipitating factors: flashing lights, lack of sleep, stress. ☐
7. Advises the patient not to go swimming alone and take showers, not baths. ☐
8. Advises the patient about increased risk of accidents. ☐
9. Advised the patient to avoid dangerous sports like rock-climbing, canoeing, skiing, scuba diving. ☐
10. Advises the patient on oral contraception: carbamazepine increases breakdown of pill and increases risk of birth defects; barrier methods recommended. ☐
11. Explains driving regulations: the patient should inform the DVLA of her diagnosis. ☐
12. To be able to drive civilian vehicles, she must be free of all seizures while awake for 1 year, or have suffered only sleeping seizures for 3 years. Rules are stricter for road haulage, piloting aeroplanes, operating heavy machinery, etc. ☐
13. Explains carbamazepine's side-effects e.g. dizziness, drowsiness, headache, rash, blurred vision, and reduced folate absorption. ☐
14. Explains carbamazepine dose gradually increases, with regular plasma level monitoring. ☐
15. Explains treatment may need to be changed or augmented. ☐
16. Explains that prognosis is good; most people are weaned off medication within 5 years. ☐
17. Mentions leaflet, website or epilepsy group, at which point examiner hands the patient a leaflet. ☐
18. Asks for questions. ☐
19. Explains that medication should not be suddenly stopped for exams as seizure risk would be more disruptive. ☐
20. Overall impression. ☐

Examiner's additional questions (near the end)

21. **Q:** (asked if driving discussed) **Should Ms White refuse to stop driving despite her diagnosis, what would you do?**
    A: Inform the Drivers and Vehicle Licensing Agency (DVLA). ☐

TOTAL SCORE / 42

Further information

People with active epilepsy have mortality rates ~3 times as high as the age-matched general population. ~20% is from **sudden unexplained death in epilepsy** (SUDEP).

Following a single seizure, 40% have a 2nd seizure within 1 year and 50% within 3 years. 70-80% of people who suffer tonic-clonic seizures can have their epilepsy controlled on 1 drug, compared to 30-40% of people with partial seizures.

After at least 2 years without seizures, gradual weaning from medication can commence, provided neurological examination and EEG is normal. Gradual dose reduction is recommended because sudden withdrawal can precipitate severe seizures. The Drivers Medical Unit of the DVLA advises that patients should not drive for 6 months after medication has ceased. The DVLA stipulates that drivers of commercial vehicles must be free of seizures and off medication for at least 10 years. Giving safety advice and documenting doing so after the diagnosis of epilepsy is very important, as doctors who fail to do this risk being held legally liable for subsequent accidents.

OSCE 14 – History

Actor instructions

You are tired, irritable and in pain. You use your left arm for gesturing, but not your right as it is weak. If candidate asks too many questions, particularly about your history of alcoholism, you loudly talk over them about your headache. You reveal more unprompted symptoms when asked open questions and not interrupted.

When asked about	You mention
Name	Hello, I'm Julia Garrison.
Headache	I've had this awful headache. It's been getting worse for about 6 or 7 weeks.
	I wake up and it's on me like a sledgehammer, that's my wake-up call, that's my alarm clock. Every day. Especially the left side of my head and it seems to move backwards from there. What can you do for me? Aspirin is nothing, paracetamol does nothing.
Alleviating factors	Nothing makes it better. Drinking can make it better if it can take my mind off it, but I hardly drink no more. I used to be into the drugs scene, the drinking scene, but I'm not on that scene no more, it's a young person's game. I'm forty-one, you know that? Does it say that on your notes? I've blacked out on the drink before, but I've hardly taking anything these days and I've blacked out twice, how do you explain that? *[Coughs]* Fuck, it hurts when I cough.
Blackouts	Well I just wake up on the floor, feeling even worse, tired, sometimes bruised. And how do you explain this *[lifts weak right arm with left then lets it drop]*? I can't handle things with my right arm. If I take a can or a cup of tea in my left arm that's going on the floor, on the carpet, no warning.
Timing	It's not something I can get away from. It's like

heavy artillery, pounding all day. I'm not keeping my food down either, puking up all sorts. I've lost about half a stone in just the last week.

If anything makes it worse

It's worse in the morning, if I lean forward it gets worse; if I lie down it gets worse; if I laugh it gets worse. I'm having no fun these days.

Severity out of 10

It's awful; nowadays it's about 10 out of 10 first thing in the morning. I've had 2 kids and this can get worse than that.

Past medical history

Well apart from the alcohol, I used to be into drugs, coke and speed and all that, but I never injected. And that was all years and years ago. I've been healthy my whole life, never even had to go to hospital before.

Medication

I've tried aspirin and paracetamol. I'm not taking the pill, I'm not taking anything.

Drinking

Like I say, I was off it for ages, maybe now I'll drink one can of cider of a morning, especially since I've been off work this last week, just one can and just because I've been feeling so shit. I work in advertising. But I'm not rattling, none of that.

Marking Scheme	
2 marks: Good - 1 mark: Adequate - 0 mark: Poor/Not done	**Mark 0 – 2**
1. Polite introduction, takes patient's name.	☐
Finds out about pain:	
2. ▪ Duration	☐
3. ▪ Character	☐
4. ▪ Radiation	☐
5. ▪ Alleviating factors	☐
6. ▪ Timing	☐

7. ▪ Exacerbating factors ☐
8. ▪ Severity ☐
9. Finds out about vomiting and weight loss.
10. Asks about drinking.
11. Asks about past medical history.
12. Asks about medication.
13. Finds out about medication.
14. Finds out about blackouts.
15. Finds out about left arm weakness.
16. Overall impression. ☐

Examiner's additional questions (near the end)

Q: What is the diagnosis?
17. **A:** Space-occupying lesion. ☐

Q: What would you expect to find on examination?
18. **A:** Lists features of space-occupying lesion e.g. focal UMN ☐
    signs, abducens nerve palsy, Cushing's sign (secondary
    hypertension and bradycardia), papilloedema.

Q: What would you do next?
19. **A:** Advises urgent admission. ☐

TOTAL SCORE **/ 38**

Further information
Primary and metastatic brain tumours each have an annual incidence in
the UK of ~8 per 100 000 people, ~10% of all solid tumours. Other causes
of space occupying lesions include abscesses, aneurysms, cysts and
subdural haemorrhages.

Space-occupying lesions lead to **signs of raised intracranial pressure**,
including hypertension and bradycardia (Cushing reflex), headache made
worse by lying down/ straining/ induced by coughing, papilloedema, seizures, false localising signs (e.g. VI nerve palsy), focal signs, irregular
(Cheyne-Stokes) breathing, reduced consciousness and vomiting.

Frontal lobe damage may cause emotional lability, expressive dysphasia (dominant side, understanding relatively intact) and contralateral UMN signs. Dominant temporal lobe damage can cause receptive dysphasia (understanding impaired).

Parietal lesion impairs touch sensation contralaterally, dominant lobe lesions can cause Gerstmann syndrome (remembered as **AALF**: **A**calculia - inability to perform mathematic calculations, **A**lexia - inability to read, **L**eft-right disorientation, **F**inger agnosia - inability to distinguish the fingers of one's own hand) while non-dominant lobe lesions can cause neglect of the contralateral visual hemifield and anosognosia, whereby hemiparesis is not acknowledged by the patient. Neglect is temporarily alleviated by injecting cold water into the ear ipsilateral to the neglected side or warm water into the contralateral ear.

Lumbar puncture is contraindicated with suspected space-occupying lesion, due to the risk of death by brainstem coning; CT scan may be required to rule this out. Other investigations include contrast MRI, mammography, chest x-ray, HIV test and brain biopsy. Ventriculo-peritoneal shunts can ease obstructive hydrocephalus, blockages occurring most commonly at the long and narrow cerebral aqueduct between the third and forth ventricles. High intracranial pressure may possibly be alleviated by sitting the patient up, IV mannitol and dexamethasone to control oedema, therapeutic hyperventilation (reducing carbon dioxide levels prevents cerebral vasodilatation) and stool softeners. Treatment is by surgery, radiotherapy and chemotherapy.

OSCE 15 – History

Actor instructions

You are fully alert and communicative; your answers are based on the responses below. You do not talk about incontinence or driving unless specifically asked, but otherwise are more likely to reveal symptoms unprompted when asked open questions and not interrupted.

When asked about	You mention
Name	Hello my name's Ronny Harris.
Presenting complaint	In the last month I've been having these proper odd episodes, 3 of them. I could tell something was going wrong because I saw flashing lights just before, like a kaleidoscope.
	One happened in school, the other 2 were at home, about an hour before I was going to bed.
Witnesses	The last time, my brer said I dropped to the floor and everyone was staring because I shouted something out.
	It was a geography class and I'm always in trouble with my teacher innit, so she was about to get vexed, that's what my friend said afterward. He said I was shaking on the floor about 3 minutes.
If anything brings them on	Nothing special brought these on, I wouldn't say I was stressed or nothing.
Loss of consciousness	Me, I just blacked out, boom, on the floor. Next thing I remember, I'm down there proper knackered, you get me? I try and get up but my arms and legs feel like lead though.
	Plus I could taste bare blood in my mouth where I bit my tongue. They let me go home after that cos all I wanted to do was sleep.
Incontinence	Yeah, I pissed myself, and that's not normal for

me. They had to lend me trousers from lost property; they were trackies so everyone knew. I didn't shit myself though.

How you feel between seizures

I'm okay between seizures, I play football, play basketball, do my homework, overstand? I'm feeling OK at the moment. I can sleep 4 or 5 hours after, then I'm pretty normal.

Previous seizures

I've never had anything like this before though.

Headache

I got a bit of a headache when I come round, but not anything else, not even a migraine.

Head injury

I've never had no head injury before.

Fever

I don't feel hot.

Medication

I'm not on any medication.

Alcohol or drug use

Me, I don't drink. Weed, that's something different, right. If I go to a party, I might smoke some spliff, but I aint done it in a month. I tried coke once, about 2 years ago and I didn't like it. I'm more interested in reading books, to be honest.

Past medical history

I've been healthy most of my life.

Family history

My older brother never had this problem; neither did anyone in my family.

Where you grew up

Round here.

Driving

I don't drive.

Marking Scheme

2 marks: Good - 1 mark: Adequate - 0 mark: Poor/Not done	Mark 0 – 2
1. Polite introduction; takes patient's name.	☐
2. Finds when funny turns started.	☐
3. Finds out about aura.	☐
4. Asks about precipitating factors.	☐
5. Finds what witness saw.	☐
6. Finds out about loss of consciousness.	☐
7. Asks about urinary and faecal incontinence.	☐
8. Finds out how he felt after the turns.	☐
9. Asks how he feels between turns.	☐
10. Asks about head injury.	☐
11. Asks about headache.	☐
12. Asks about fever.	☐
13. Asks about previous history of seizures.	☐
14. Asks about drug history.	☐
15. Asks about alcohol and drug use.	☐
16. Asks about past medical history.	☐
17. Asks about family history.	☐
18. Asks about driving.	☐
19. Explains epilepsy driving restrictions for civilian vehicles- must be fit-free 1 year with waking seizures, 3 years for sleeping seizures. Stricter rules for lorries and planes.	☐
20. Thanks the patient. Overall impression.	☐

Examiner's additional questions (near the end)

Q: What is your provisional diagnosis?	
21. A: Generalized tonic-clonic seizures caused by idiopathic epilepsy.	☐
Q: What investigations would you recommend?	
22. A: Recommends 5+ appropriate investigations:- FBC, U&E, LFT, serum calcium and phosphate, blood glucose, drug screen, ECG, CT, lumbar puncture, EEG.	☐

TOTAL SCORE — / 44

Further information
Epilepsy has ~1% prevalence, and is diagnosed following a minimum of 2 seizures. Generalized seizures stem from diffuse abnormal brain activity and impair consciousness. Simple partial seizures stem from focal activity and do not impair consciousness, while complex partial seizures are focal but impair consciousness.

Secondary generalized seizures begin with focal activity which becomes generalized. Generalized seizures include tonic-clonic, absence, myo-clonic, tonic (increased rigidity without convulsions) and atonic (flaccidity alone) seizures. Epileptic seizures can occur in any individual by drugs or metabolic abnormalities which reduce the seizure threshold. Seizures are more likely in epileptic people with stress, sleep deprivation, non-concordance to medication, when drinking alcohol or when exposed to strobe lighting. When an adult has a suspected seizure, a detailed clinical history and examination is performed. More than 50% of people with epilepsy will have non-diagnostic EEG's when tested, but a positive result, which can be provoked by sleep deprivation, photic stimulation or hyperventilation, has a high diagnostic value. ECG may be needed to investigate cardiogenic causes of syncope, which can be mistaken for seizures. CT or MRI may be required to rule out brain lesions.

Due to safety restrictions, it is important to ask about driving and to document the advice given. If the doctor does not explain these to the patient and they have an accident, the doctor is legally liable. For a full list of safety advice measures, see OSCE 13.

OSCE 16 – History

Actor instructions
You are frightened and upset, with a severe headache; your neck is stiff and painful to move. If they ask too many questions, you get annoyed but if they ask open questions and do not interrupt, you speak more easily.

When asked about	You mention
Name	Hello I'm Loretta Partridge.
Headache	I've been getting migraines since I was 13. Today about half an hour ago I was helping my mum in the garden when this headache come on like someone hit the back of me head with a cricket bat. It's terrible, worse than my migraines. I've vomited since then and still feel sick.
Movement	It doesn't seem to move anywhere, but it hurts when I move my neck.
Alleviating factors	Nothing seems to make it better. [When asked about timing]: It's been constant for the last half hour, not getting worse or any better.
Severity out of 10	I'd say this was a 10 out of 10, it couldn't get worse, except maybe when I cough. The paramedic made me laugh on the way here; that made it worse too. I've never had more pain in my life. I can't even look at the lights because it hurts my eyes.
Family history	I don't know my grandparents or my dad. I've not heard of anyone having this problem.
Medication	I'm not on anything. I tried taking aspirin and paracetamol, but they weren't any use. Is there anything stronger I could have?
Fever	I don't have a temperature; my mum took it and said it was normal.

Rash   I don't have a rash.

Past medical   I've always been healthy.
history

Marking Scheme	
2 marks: Good - 1 mark: Adequate - 0 mark: Poor/Not done	**Mark** **0 – 2**

1. Polite introduction; takes patient's name. ☐
2. Finds duration of headache ☐
    Finds out about pain:
3. ▪ Character ☐
4. ▪ Radiation ☐
5. ▪ Alleviating factors ☐
6. ▪ Timing ☐
7. ▪ Exacerbating factors ☐
8. ▪ Severity ☐
9. Finds out about history of migraine. ☐
10. Asks about family history. ☐
11. Asks about medication. ☐
12. Finds out about neck stiffness and photophobia. ☐
13. Asks about fever. ☐
14. Asks about rash. ☐
15. Finds out about vomiting. ☐
16. Asks about past medical history. ☐
17. Overall impression. ☐

Examiner's additional questions (near the end)

Q: What is your diagnosis?
18. **A:** Subarachnoid haemorrhage ☐

Q: What is your immediate management?
19. **A:** Mentions need for analgesia, anti-emetics. ☐
20. **A:** Recommends that her airway, breathing and circulation
    are monitored, and that she be sat up and given oxygen, ☐

TOTAL SCORE   **/ 40**

Further information

Subarachnoid haemorrhage (SAH) is an arterial bleed into the cerebrospinal fluid between the arachnoid and pia mater, risk factors include collagen disorders (e.g. Ehler-Danlos syndrome, polycystic kidneys), smoking, hypertension (exacerbated by cocaine use). Causes include rupture of berry aneurysms (~80% of cases) and angiomas (~5% of cases); mycotic aneurysms are caused by bacterial infection of artery walls.

Berry aneurysms can affect the anterior cerebral artery (35%-40% of cases), the internal carotid (~30%), the middle cerebral artery (20-25%) and the posterior circulation (~10%). Incidence is 5-10 per 100 000 people per year, and it causes a severe sudden-onset headache, often described as "thunderclap", alongside meningism (neck stiffness, photophobia, Brudzinski's and Kernig's signs) and raised intracranial pressure.

Urgent contrast CT (recent haemorrhage appears white) is required. Lumbar punctures can detect haemorrhages that CT misses, showing xanthochromia (yellow tinge) and raised red cell count hours after the haemorrhage.

Urgent neurosurgery is often required (e.g. clipping or non-invasive radiological guided coil embolization), with control of intracranial hypertension, (sitting the patient up, therapeutic hyperventilation to prevent vasodilatation, IV mannitol and stool softeners to prevent straining may help), prevention of cerebral vasoconstriction using nimodipine (calcium channel antagonist), blood pressure control (minimise risk of re-bleed while maintaining adequate perfusion). SAH can obstruct CSF drainage and cause hydrocephalus, for which ventricular shunts may be required. SAH prognosis is poor, nearly 50% die within hours and up to 20% more within weeks.

Survivors require neuropsychological evaluation to gauge functional impairment. With SAH excluded, meningitis, space-occupying lesion, sinus thrombosis and migraine are possible diagnoses.

OSCE 17 – History

Actor instructions

You are in pain and irritable. You reveal more unprompted information when asked open questions and not interrupted, though some elements, like features of intracranial pressure have to be specifically asked about.

When asked about	You mention
Name	Hello I'm Lavine Taylor.
Presenting complaint	About 2 months ago I started getting these really bad pounding headaches. Really relentless, they make me nauseous. I can't concentrate at work and I've been home early a few times, told my sister to look after my kids and keep them quiet.
Movement	It starts around my temples but spreads all over my head.
What makes the headaches better	Normally if I can have some aspirin and rest, that helps, just somewhere dark and quiet.
Timing	I know when it's coming on maybe half an hour beforehand, because I start seeing shapes and lines flashing up.
What makes the headaches worse	It hurts to cough sometimes, and they come on after I've eaten chocolate sometimes, or cheese. I think they're worse when I'm stressed up, like in the supermarket the other day when my youngest was mucking around.
Severity out of 10	I'd say it was 6 out of 10.
Medication	I'm on no medication apart from aspirin, paracetamol and the oral contraceptive pill.
When you started the oral contraceptive pill	I started it about 3 months ago.

If pain is worse when lying down/in morning/laughing	When the pain comes on, I go to sleep if I can and that makes it better. It comes on at any time, not necessarily the morning.
Motor or sensory symptoms	Other than these bursts, which last hours, I'm not permanently affected.
Fever	I don't have a fever or anything like that. When I've not got these headaches, I feel fine.
Past medical history	I've been deaf in my right ear since I was a kid, but otherwise I'm fine.
Family history	No one in my family has headaches like this.
If you have any questions	Do you think this could be a brain tumour?

Marking Scheme

2 marks: Good - 1 mark: Adequate - 0 mark: Poor/Not done — Mark 0 – 2

1. Polite introduction; takes patient's name.
2. Finds duration of headache.
    Finds out about pain:
3. ▪ Character
4. ▪ Radiation
5. ▪ Alleviating factors
6. ▪ Timing
7. ▪ Exacerbating factors
8. ▪ Severity
9. Finds out about vomiting.
10. Finds out about prodrome visual disturbance.
11. Excludes other symptoms such as morning headache, focal signs, fever.
12. Asks about previous history of headache.
13. Asks about family history.

14. Asks her if she has any questions, reassures her brain tumour is unlikely, far rarer than migraine, which her symptoms resemble. ☐
15. Thanks the patient. Overall impression. ☐

Examiner's additional questions (near the end)

Q: What is your diagnosis and why?
16. **A:** Migraine, triggered by cheese and chocolate, oral contraceptive pill use, preceding visual prodrome with no focal signs, no seizures, good general health. ☐

17. **Q: What is the management?**
A: Suggests suitable treatment, e.g. propranolol or pizotifen for prevention, aspirin, paracetamol or sumatriptan and antiemetics for acute attack. ☐

TOTAL SCORE / 34

Further information

Migraine is a common form (~10% lifetime prevalence) of recurrent throbbing headache, classified as with or without aura. Precipitating factors include stress, consuming cheese, red wine or chocolate, premenstrual hormone levels, pregnancy and oral contraceptive pill use.

Migraine has been proposed to be caused by meningeal vessel vasoconstriction, followed by prolonged overcompensating and painful vasodilatation. Migraine prophylactics include vasodilators (e.g. propranolol) and acute treatment includes vasoconstrictors (e.g. sumatriptan 5- HT_1 agonist). Migraine with aura involves transient prodromal symptoms, such as flashing lights (teichopsia), jagged lines (fortification spectra), tingling, hemiparesis (rare) and weakness.

The commoner migraine without aura involves less defined visual prodromes, but similar headache and nausea. The headache can be unilateral or generalised, tending to last several hours. Treatment involves mild analgesics like tolfenamic acid, paracetamol and sometimes anti-emetics like metoclopramide. Avoidance of triggers and quitting smoking may also help. Tension headache has been attributed to nerve irritation and scalp muscle tension, causing throbbing tightness and eye pressure. It can be difficult to differentiate from migraine and responds to treatment with anti-migraine drugs, antidepressants, ice packs and massage.

Cluster headaches are unilateral and intense, affecting men ~5 times more commonly than women, recurrent pain tending to focus around the eye. This can last hours and causes lacrimation, nasal congestion and vomiting. It rarely responds to standard analgesics, but can be treated by subcutaneous sumatriptan injection ($5HT_1$ agonist) and therapeutic hyper-ventilation (100% oxygen at 7-12 litres per minute), with possible lithium prophylaxis.

OSCE 18 – Consent for lumbar puncture

Actor instructions
You are feverish and in discomfort, but can understand and retain information.

When asked about	You mention
Your name	Hello, I'm Tariq Achebe.
Current situation	I came in here with a bad headache and a fever. The GP gave me an injection of the antibiotics before I got here and I've been on a drip. I feel nauseous, weak and still very ill. The nurse told me I need a spinal tap. I don't know what this is or why it is needed.
If you have any questions	If you don't do the lumbar puncture, will you still be able to treat me?

Marking Scheme	
2 marks: Good - 1 mark: Adequate - 0 mark: Poor/Not done	**Mark 0 – 2**
1. Polite introduction, verifies patient's identity.	☐
2. Finds out about current clinical situation.	☐
3. Explains why lumbar puncture is indicated (to sample cerebrospinal fluid, in which the brain and spinal cord float).	☐
4. Explains that CT showed no mass, so lumbar puncture is safe.	☐
Explains procedure:	
5. ▪ Patient lies on his left side with knees bent up to chest	☐
6. ▪ Target area is marked on back- below end of spinal cord (L4 level at iliac crests in adults)	☐
7. ▪ Doctor washes their hands, puts on gloves and mask and uses sterile equipment	☐
8. ▪ Target area sterilized with iodine	☐
9. ▪ Surrounding area covered by sterile sheets	☐
10. ▪ Local anaesthetic injected- may be painful	☐
11. ▪ Needle pierces skin, spinal ligaments, dura and arachnoid layers to extract fluid	☐

12. ▪ Less than 10ml in total taken in 3 small bottles ☐
13. ▪ Dressing applied, patient remains in bed for over an hour ☐
14. Explains that complications – headache and pain at the site – are likely but short-lived. ☐
15. Asks for questions and answers competently e.g. we can continue to treat you presumptively for the most common bacterial infections, but there may be other causes which would be missed without a lumbar puncture, such as tuberculosis. If you have meningitis, this could also affect how we treat your close contacts. ☐
16. Checks understanding and asks for consent in non-directive fashion. ☐
17. Overall impression ☐

Examiner's additional questions (near the end)

Q: What are the contraindications of lumbar puncture?
18. **A:** Skin infection in lumbar region, raised intracranial pressure, clotting disorder. ☐

TOTAL SCORE **/ 36**

Further information
Lumbar puncture enables measurement of CSF pressure as well as glucose and protein levels, electrophoresis (for oligoclonal bands in MS), serology (e.g. syphilis or toxoplasmosis), microscopy, culture for organisms and their antimicrobial sensitivities, histopathological assessment (cytology) and other agents (e.g. LDH). The height of the bed should be adjusted to allow the best access. The target area, through the intervertebral spaces between L3 and L4 or L4 and L5, is located by drawing a line between the iliac crests, which are level with L4. On piercing the subarachnoid space, the opening pressure is noted. If headache after lumbar puncture is particularly severe, a "blood patch" may be performed, whereby 20ml of the patient's blood is injected into the epidural space, where it clots and seals the hole. Valid consent for a procedure requires that the patient understands what it entails, knows the risks involved and makes their choice without coercion. Competence of a patient to consent entails that the patient can understand and retain the information, weigh up its pros and cons and communicate their wishes.

OSCE 19 – History

Actor instructions
Your right eye is itchy and you occasionally rub it. You reveal more un-prompted symptoms when asked open questions and not interrupted.

When asked about	You mention
Your name	I'm Marcus Redding
Presenting complaint	My right eye's been really sticky and itchy since I woke up. It's been bothering me all day. I wouldn't describe it as a pain as such, more just itchy and uncomfortable.
Discharge	There's this yellow stuff coming out my right eye which I have to dab with tissue.
What makes the pain worse	My Nan says not to rub it because that just makes it worse, but I've been doing that anyway.
What makes the pain better	I washed my contacts, and I try and wipe away the discharge, but it's not helping.
Previous eye problems	I started wearing glasses for short-sightedness when I was twelve, ten years ago. I've been wearing contacts for six months. I've never had anything like this.
Past medical history	I've never been to hospital, hardly ever have to come to the GP normally.
Thyroid disease	No, I don't have that, not that I'm aware of.
Contact lenses	I've been wearing them for six months now, I'm short-sighted, and everyone says they make me look better. They're monthly disposables and I take them off at night and clean them using the fluid like I'm meant to.
Medication	I tried taking some aspirin, but nothing else.

Allergies   I don't have any food or drug allergies as such.

Family history   My dad, my granddad and my uncle have all had heart attacks. Both my parents wear glasses, but they're just short-sighted, nothing serious.

Marking Scheme	
2 marks: Good - 1 mark: Adequate - 0 mark: Poor/Not done	**Mark 0 – 2**
1. Polite introduction, verifies patient's name.	☐
2. Finds presenting complaint- itchy, inflamed right eye and blurred vision.	☐
3. Finds out duration.	
4. Finds out exacerbating factors and alleviating factors.	☐
5. Asks about discharge.	
6. Asks about previous eye problems.	
7. Asks about contact lens use- how often he removes them, how often he cleans them.	☐
8. Asks about past medical history.	☐
9. Asks specifically about a history of hyperthyroidism.	☐
10, Asks about medication.	☐
11. Asks about allergies.	☐
12. Asks about family history.	☐
13. Thanks the patient. Overall impression.	☐
Examiner's additional questions (near the end)	
Q: What is your diagnosis? 14. A: Bacterial conjunctivitis.	☐
Q: What is the treatment? 15. A: Antibiotic eyedrops e.g. chloramphenicol saline irrigation and advice on eye hygiene.	☐
TOTAL SCORE	**/ 30**

Further information
Symptoms of conjunctivitis are often described as discomfort, irritation or grittiness. Pain and photophobia tend to indicate more serious diagnoses such as uveitis, orbital cellulitis, keratitis, acute glaucoma and even meningitis. The likeliest causes of red painful eyes are allergy, infection and thyroid eye disease. Infective causes of conjunctivitis tend become bilateral due to rubbing, causing a purulent discharge with crusting, while corneal abrasions, viral and atopic conjunctivitis cause watery discharge. Iritis, glaucoma and atopic conjunctivitis are generally bilateral.

Recent upper respiratory tract infections may lead to adenovirus conjunctivitis, which can occur in epidemics. Herpes simplex can cause retinitis, blepharitis, conjunctivitis, iritis and keratitis, with recurrence on viral reactivation in the trigeminal ganglia and is one of the commonest causes of corneal blindness in the world. It is treated with oral or topical aciclovir. Allergic conjunctivitis is particularly characterised by an atopic history and strong itching; it is treated with antihistamine eye drops.

Bacterial conjunctivitis is suggested above by the **unilateral onset**, **contact lens use** and **purulent discharge**. The commonest causes of bacterial conjunctivitis are Staphylococcus Aureus, Haemophilus Influenza and Streptococcus Pneumoniae; though infection tends to be self-limiting, duration, complications and infectiousness can be reduced by a short course of antibiotic eye-drops, such as chloramphenicol.

N. Gonorrhoea, N. Meningitidis and C. Trachomatis cause serious bacterial conjunctivitis, presenting in neonates or sexually active adults with bilateral purulent discharge. Without treatment, it may progress to corneal ulceration and perforation, with disseminated infection possible in neonates. Investigations include cell cultures, polymerase chain reaction and monoclonal antibody staining. Treatment involves IV and eye-drop ceftriaxone, saline irrigation and advice on eye hygiene.

OSCE 20 – Examination

Note for the examiner:
Tell the candidate to move on before performing unpleasant tests such as gag and corneal reflexes, asking them only to explain.

Marking Scheme	
2 marks: Good - 1 mark: Adequate - 0 mark: Poor/Not done	**Mark 0 – 2**
1. Polite introduction, explains what they will do, gains consent.	☐
2. Washes their hands.	☐
3. Asks about pain before starting.	☐
4. Clearly inspects patient from the end of the bed.	☐
5. **I:** Asks about any recent change in smell. Explains they could test further by smell recognition.	☐
6. **II:** Tests each eye's acuity individually with Snellen chart (while wearing spectacles/ contacts) positioned 6m away, mentions would like to test colour vision.	☐
7. Tests visual fields in each eye using pen (removes patient's glasses first).	☐
8. Tests direct and consensual light reflexes, looking for relative afferent pupillary defect with swinging light test.	☐
9. Tests for accommodation reflex.	☐
10. **III, IV, VI:** Tests eye motion tracking a finger moving in the pattern of an 'H', looking for dysconjugate gaze and pausing to check for nystagmus at ~30° deviation from central.	☐
11. **V:** Sensory: Mentions they would normally test pain and temperature, but won't in this case.	☐
12. Fine touch: Starts with a proximal test e.g. on the sternum.	☐
13. Tests ophthalmic (**V1**), maxillary (**V2**) and mandibular (**V3**) dermatomes bilaterally using a piece of rolled cotton with the patient's eyes closed. Asks if it feels the same as on the sternum and on either side.	☐
14. Explains they would normally perform the corneal reflex (tests V (afferent) and VII (efferent)).	☐
15. **V:** Motor: Asks the patient to clench their teeth while they feel temporalis and masseter.	☐

16. Asks the patient to open their mouth and keep it open while they try to close it (lateral pterygoid strength). ☐
17. Tests jaw jerk reflex. ☐
    VII: Motor: Instructs the patient to:
18. ▪ Screw up their eyes (orbicularis oculi), smile (risorius) ☐
19. ▪ Blow out their cheeks (orbicularis oris), raise their eye brows (occipitofrontalis) ☐
20. VII: Taste: Asks about changes in taste. ☐
21. VIII: Screens hearing e.g. whispering a number into one ear while rubbing fingers together near other ear, then asking the patient to repeat back. ☐
22. Weber's test: places the vibrating tuning fork in the midline of the patient's forehead and asks them if it is heard louder in either ear. ☐
23. Rinné's test: places the vibrating tuning fork on the mastoid process and asks the patient to say when they no longer hear the vibrations. Then moves it next to the external auditory meatus and asks if it is audible. ☐
24. Balance: Romberg test: asks patient to stand upright with their feet together. Observes for unsteadiness, reassures them that they will be caught, asks them to close their eyes, observing again. ☐
25. IX, X: Asks patient to say 'ah' and watches the soft palate using a torch if available. ☐
26. Explains they would gently test posterior pharynx sensation. ☐
27. Explains they would ask them to sip a glass of water and watch for regurgitation. ☐
28. XI: Asks patient to shrug shoulders and to resist light pres sure being exerted on them (trapezius). ☐
29. Asks patient to turn their head against resistance while feeling contralateral neck muscle (sternomastoid). ☐
30. XII: Asks patient to stick out tongue and bend it to either side ☐
31. Thanks the patient, Overall impression. ☐

Examiner's additional questions (near the end)

Q: To which side does the mandible deviate with a unilateral V lesion?
32. **A:** Mandible deviates towards side of V lesion. ☐

Q: To which side does the uvula deviate with a
unilateral X lesion?

33. A: Uvula deviates away from side of X lesion. ☐

Q: To which side does the tongue deviate with a
unilateral XII lesion?

34. A: Tongue deviates towards side of XII lesion. ☐

TOTAL SCORE | **/ 68**

Further information
Normally, each pupil should constrict when individually illuminated (direct
light reflex) and when light reaches the contralateral eye (consensual light
reflex), due to decussating afferent and efferent fibers. Paradoxical dilatation occurs in the swinging light test of **optic (II)** and **oculomotor (III)**
nerves when the pupil dilates on direct illumination, due to II lesions (relative afferent pupillary defect) making the consensual reflex stronger than
the direct. Causes of relative afferent pupillary defect (Marcus-Gunn pupil)
include multiple sclerosis, neurosyphilis, giant cell arteritis, glaucoma, unilateral optic nerve compression and unilateral retinal damage. By conven-
tion, acuity is tested with spectacles/ contacts on because refractive errors
are not due to cranial nerve damage.

The 4 components of the optic nerve examination can remembered by the mnemonic **AFRO**, standing for **A**cuity, **F**ields, **Re**-
flexes, **O**phthalmoscopy. III nerve innervates the iris, the levator palpe-
brae superioris (opens the eye), inferior oblique, superior rectus, inferior
rectus and medial rectus ocular muscles. The superior oblique is innervated by **trochlear (IV)** nerve (enables looking down and out) and the lateral rectus by **abducens (VI)** nerve (enables looking outwards). Accommodation is tested by asking the patient to focus on a distant then a near
object, whereupon both pupils should constrict.

Nystagmus is an unintentional flickering eye movement featuring slow
tracking followed by fast correction in the opposite direction. Nystagmus
occurs with damage to **III, IV, VI, VIII**, cerebellum or brainstem (vertical
nystagmus). Fine nystagmus is physiological at the extreme peripheries of
vision. Damage along the III sympathetic pathway from the midbrain passing the cervical spinal cord (e.g. syringomyelia), sympathetic chain (e.g.
carotid artery dissection) and apical lung (e.g. lung cancer) results in

Horner's syndrome, featuring miosis (constricted pupil), ptosis (drooping eyelid), loss of sweating above the eyebrow (anhydrosis), and enophthalmos (eye appears sunken).

The **trigeminal (V)** nerve enables touch sensation for the face, conjunctivae, mouth and anterior 2/3 of the tongue. The corneal reflex is tested by touching the cornea with cotton wool rolled to a point, which normally causes the eye to shut, requiring intact **V1** and **VII** nerves. The **V** motor component supplies the muscles of mastication (temporalis, masseter, medial and lateral pterygoids) which have bilateral cortical innervation, thus unilateral UMN **V** lesions don't produce motor signs.

The **facial nerve (VII)** sensory component is responsible for taste from the anterior 2/3 of the tongue, while its motor component controls facial expression and the stapedius muscle of the middle ear. Upper facial muscles, like the occipitofrontalis, have bilateral UMN innervation, meaning their function remains intact following a contralateral UMN lesion. **Bell's phenomenon** occurs with LMN **VII** palsy at the orbicularis oculi whereby the eye can't be closed fully, leaving the white of the eye partially exposed. **Ramsay-Hunt syndrome** is a form of shingles, causing vesicle formation in the ear and **VII** LMN palsy.

The **vestibulocochlear (VIII)** nerve enables hearing and balance. **Rinné's test** is positive if the patient can hear the fork when it is placed at the external auditory meatus (normal). A conductive hearing loss is suggested when the fork can be heard from the mastoid but not when placed at the meatus (Rinné negative). A person with sensorineural but no conductive defect would be equally impaired whether it was placed at the mastoid or the meatus.

With **Weber's test**, the tuning fork is heard more clearly on the side of a pure conductive hearing loss because vibrations are more weakly transmitted to the cochlea via the external and middle ear, reducing destructive interference with signals travelling via the skull bones. With pure sensorineural loss, the fork is heard more strongly in the unaffected ear.

The **W**eber test can be remembered by the fork on someone's forehead can make them look like a **W**ally, while "**Rinné**" sounds similar to "**ringing**", which is what the fork does by the meatus. **Romberg test** is positive when the patient becomes more unsteady with their eyes closed, suggesting **VIII**, cerebellar or proprioceptive dysfunction.

The **glossopharyngeal (IX)** supplies motor function to the parotid glands and receives taste and touch input from the posterior 1/3 of the tongue and sensation from the posterior pharynx. Gag reflex tests **IX** sensory and **X** motor function, but isn't necessary when uvula movement is inspected and sensation of the posterior pharynx can be tested. **Bulbar palsy** is a LMN lesion of **IX, X** and **XII**. **Pseudobulbar palsy** is a bilateral UMN lesion of the same nerves. The **hypoglossal (XII)** nerve innervates the tongue musculature, palsy causes wasting, fasciculation and tongue deviation towards the affected side. The **accessory (XI)** nerve controls the trapezius (enables shoulder abduction) and sternocleidomastoid (enables head rotation towards the contralateral side) muscles.

Causes of specific combined cranial nerve palsies include thrombosis/tumour/ aneurysm of the lateral sinus (**VI and VII**), cavernous sinus (**III, IV, V1 and VI**) or inferior petrosal sinus (**V and VI**), jugular foramen lesions (**IX, X, XI**), motor neurone disease (**IX, X, XII**), syringobulbia (**III, V, VII, IX, X**), lateral medullary syndrome (**III, V, VIII, IX, X**- causes dissociated pain and temperature loss on ipsilateral side of face and contralateral side of body and limbs) and cerebellopontine angle lesions (**V, VII, VIII**). Other multiple deficits are seen with diffuse brainstem injury, Guillain-Barré syndrome, mononeuritis multiplex and trauma. The cranial nerves can be recalled using the mnemonic "**O**n **O**ld **O**lympus **T**owering **T**ops, **A** **F**inn **A**nd **G**erman **V**iewed **S**ome **H**ops" (Gupta 1998), though there are dirtier versions.

9   Psychiatry OSCEs

OSCE 1 – History [5 minutes]
(See page 197 for actor's brief and marking scheme)

You are a medical student at an outpatients' clinic. Please take a history from a 25-year-old woman with a skin problem.

OSCE 2 – History [5 minutes]
(See page 201 for actor's brief and marking scheme)

You are a medical student at a Drug Dependency Unit. Please take a substance abuse history from the following 28-year-old patient.

OSCE 3 – History [5 minutes]
(See page 205 for actor's brief and marking scheme)

You are a medical student attending a psychiatry outpatient clinic. Take a history from Mrs Jean Howie, 42, who has reported feeling tense and nervy. You will be asked for a diagnosis and to briefly explain treatment options.

OSCE 4 – Explaining ECT [5 minutes]
(See page 208 for actor's brief and marking scheme)

Ms Janine Adams has severe depression that is not responding to drug treatment. She has been recommended for electroconvulsive therapy (ECT); explain the procedure with a view to gaining valid consent.

Indication: severe depression not responding to drugs.

Procedure: Patient is nil by mouth for at least 8 hours. They are rendered unconscious with a rapid-acting general anaesthetic that lasts about 5 minutes, muscle relaxants are given, and an electric current is applied to the right side of the head. 2 electrodes are placed 10cm away from each other, one above the ear, one between the eye and the ear. The current is applied for 15 seconds, inducing muscle contraction followed by a tonic clonic seizure, lasting about 1 minute. Then they are placed in the recovery position and monitored until they regain consciousness. In case of arrhythmias, resuscitation equipment is available. In case of agitation on recovery, midazolam is ready for injection. Treatment consists of 6 sessions over 3 weeks.

Side effects: some loss of short-term memory, possible agitation, headache, nausea and vomiting, temporary confusion, risk of arrhythmias, anaesthetic complications. Good safety record overall.

Contraindications: Recent subdural/ subarachnoid haemorrhage, any contraindication to general anaesthesia.

Cautions: recent stroke, myocardial infarct, arrhythmias.

OSCE 5 – History [5 minutes]
(See page 211 for actor's brief and marking scheme)

You are a medical student attending a psychiatry outpatient clinic. Take a history from the next patient, Mr Vikesh Kambli, 35. You will be asked for a diagnosis and to briefly explain treatment options.

OSCE 6 – History [5 minutes]
(See page 217 for actor's brief and marking scheme)

You are a medical student attending a General Practice; please take a history from Mrs Marie Jenkins, 32, with a view to making a diagnosis.

OSCE 7 – Written station [5 minutes]
(See page 221 for answers)

Ms BH weighs 40kg and has a height of 5 foot 4 inches, what is her body mass index? 1 inch = 2.54 cm (1 mark)
What are the 4 ICD-10 defining features of anorexia nervosa? What are the other clinical features? (8 marks)
Give 3 risk factors for anorexia nervosa. (3 marks)
Give 3 relevant investigations for anorexia nervosa (3 marks)
List medical complications of anorexia nervosa. (3 marks)
List the treatment modalities. (2 marks)

OSCE 8 – Clozapine treatment [5 minutes]
(See page 223 for actor's brief and marking scheme)

Mr John Ferris has schizophrenia and agreed to start treatment with clozapine. Read the information below and explain it to Mr Ferris.

Indication: schizophrenia inadequately controlled despite the sequential use of 2 or more antipsychotics (one of which should be an atypical antipsychotic) each for at least 6-8 weeks (NICE 2002).

Side-effects
- Blood disorders: neutropenia, agranulocytosis therefore must report any sign of infection, like a fever or sore throat, immediately.
- Cardiovascular: postural hypotension, myocarditis (most common in first 2 months), cardiomyopathy, tachycardia, hypertension.
- Gastrointestinal: weight gain, constipation, sialorrhoea, nausea and vomiting, hepatitis.
- Neurological: dizziness, tardive dyskinesia, blurred vision, headache, tremor, rigidity.

Cautions: liver impairment, renal impairment, prostatic hypertrophy, angle-closure glaucoma (BNF).

Contraindications: severe heart disease, acute liver disease, severe renal impairment, history of neutropenia or agranulocytosis, paralytic ileus, bone marrow disorders, alcoholic and toxic psychoses, history of circulatory collapse, coma or severe CNS depression, drug intoxication, pregnancy, breast feeding (BNF)

Clozaril patient monitoring service: Patient, prescriber and pharmacist need to be registered. Medical history, physical examination, weight, blood pressure, FBC, LFT, lipid profile, fasting blood glucose and ECG are required before starting clozapine. After this, weekly FBC's for at 18 weeks, then at least every 2 weeks, then, if stable after 1 year, every 4 weeks and 4 weeks after terminating treatment. Blood pressure, weight and LFT must also be monitored.

OSCE 9 – Explaining autism [5 minutes]
(See page 225 for actor's brief and marking scheme)

Mrs Gina Desmond's son Jeffrey has been diagnosed with autism. Explain to her what this means, what support is available and take her questions.

OSCE 10 – Mental test score [5 minutes]
(See page 228 for actor's brief and marking scheme)

Mrs Agnes Bellman has been brought to you by her relatives, who say that she is confused. Perform an abbreviated mental test score on her.

OSCE 11 – Explaining schizophrenia [5 minutes]
(See page 230 for actor's brief and marking scheme)

Mrs Lisa Rutherford's brother has recently been diagnosed with schizophrenia; please explain to her what this means and the treatment that is available.

OSCE 12 – History [5 minutes]
(See page 233 for actor's brief and marking scheme)

Mr John Randolph, 18, is a psychiatric inpatient. Please take a history from him with a view to making a diagnosis.

OSCE 13 – History [5 minutes]
(See page 238 for actor's brief and marking scheme)

Mr Kurdt Fraser, 29, is a psychiatric patient managed in the community. Please take a history from him with a view to making a diagnosis.

OSCE 14 – Mental health act [5 minutes]
(See page 241 for actor's brief and marking scheme)

You are a junior doctor working on-call during a psychiatric rotation. A GP phones you regarding a disturbed patient and proceeds to ask you about the mental health act. Listen to his case history and together decide on the best course of action.

OSCE 15 – Explaining lithium treatment [5 minutes]
(See page 244 for actor's brief and marking scheme)

Gina Headley, 23, has agreed to commence maintenance treatment of her bipolar disorder with lithium. Read the information below, explain lithium treatment to her and ask for her informed consent.

Lithium carbonate (BNF)

Indication: Treatment and prophylaxis of mania, prophylaxis of bipolar disorder, prophylaxis of recurrent unipolar depression. For once-daily use, may take up to 6 weeks to cause intended effects. If patient responds, treatment tends to be for a minimum of 12 months.

Side-effects:
- Polyuria, polydipsia, GI disturbance, weight gain, oedema, metallic taste, fine tremor, tiredness, fetal heart deformities.

- Lithium intoxication- worsening GI disturbance, increased neurological effects (coarse tremor, blurred vision, ataxia, increasing drowsiness, dysarthria) - requires withdrawal of treatment.

- Severe overdose- convulsions, renal failure, goitre and hypothyroidism, coma, hypokalaemia, arrhythmias, circulatory failure.

Precautions:
- Before starting- thyroid, liver and renal function tests, full blood count, blood glucose, lipid profile, blood pressure, smoking and alcohol history, weight and height checks.

- During therapy- thyroid and renal function test every 6 months, serum lithium concentration every 3 months, yearly weight, height, smoking, alcohol, blood pressure and blood glucose checks. Reliable contraception is needed because of damaging effects on the foetus. Withdraw gradually if possible. Beware of signs of overdose. Beware drug interactions, especially sodium-depleting diuretics. Avoid in renal impairment, pregnancy and breast-feeding, not prescribed to children.

Lithium red card: Available from pharmacy, with information on how to take it, what to do if they miss a dose and side-effects.

OSCE 16 – History [5 minutes]
(See page 247 for actor's brief and marking scheme)

You are a medical student attending a general practice. Take a history from the Ms Waheeda Qureishi, 32, with a view to making a diagnosis.

OSCE 17 – Fitness to plead [5 minutes]
(See page 251 for actor's brief and marking scheme)

Ken Larkins, a 25-year-old man with learning difficulties, has been charged with assault and remanded in custody with a court appearance due tomorrow. The man he allegedly injured received treatment in accident and emergency but was not admitted. Determine if Mr Larkins is fit to plead.

OSCE 18 – Discussing antidepressant therapy [5 minutes]
(See page 254 for actor's brief and marking scheme)

Richard Harmon, 50, meets the ICD-10 criteria for moderate depressive disorder but is reluctant to start medication. Explore his beliefs about depression and discuss the basics of treatment, not in relation to any specific drug.

OSCE 19 – History [5 minutes]
(See page 257 for actor's brief and marking scheme)

You are a house officer who has been asked to see Belinda Robertson, 33, a patient admitted to the accident and emergency department following a suicide attempt. Please assess this patient's suicidal intent.

OSCE 20 – History [5 minutes]
(See page 260 for actor's brief and marking scheme)

You are a medical student at a psychiatric outpatients' department. Kelly Weaver, 39, has been referred by her GP feeling very low. Take a history from her with a view to reaching a diagnosis

10 | Psychiatry OSCEs Actor's brief & marking scheme

OSCE 1 – History

Actor instructions
You are a little nervous. You reveal more unprompted information when asked open questions and not interrupted.

When asked about	You mention
Your name	Hello I am Jessica Symonds.
What is wrong	I have itchy, flaky skin.
How long this has been a problem	For months, I keep washing my hands but it doesn't seem to help. Do you think they're infected?
How often you wash your hands	It's been getting worse. The other day at work I had to do it about 20 times. I realise that's excessive but if I stop myself, I get really anxious. It's like I can feel my skin getting colonized by bacteria and viruses. It makes me a lot more nervous about going out. I haven't been seeing my friends. My mother's always on at me to get help. The amount of time and energy I'm putting into it, I can't do anything else properly. I have to make excuses at work and I don't think they believe me.
The duration of the problem	I've always been into keeping things clean and germ-free, people always say how tidy my flat is. It's probably more than a year I've been washing my hands like this, but it's been getting worse in the last 3 or 4 months.

Your routines	When I wash my hands, it normally lasts 2 or 3 minutes. The water has to be hot. I collect about 4 or 5 paper towels first if it's in a public toilet. If there's a soap dispenser, I push it with my left elbow and use the tissues to turn on the taps, first I wash my palms, then my fingertips then the webbing between my fingers, then my thumbs, then the backs of my hands, then my wrists.

I do this 6 times before I feel clean. Then I turn off the taps with my elbows and dry my hands with the towels, starting with my right hand, between the fingers, then the palm, then the back of the hand then the wrist, and then my left hand.

If I accidentally touch anything dirty like the bin when I'm throwing away the towels, I have to start again.

I need to have towels left at the end to open the door; otherwise I have to wait for someone to come in for me to leave without touching the handle. If it's a push door I can just kick it.

I clean my flat every day, it can take 2 hours. |
The effect on your hands	My hands get raw, they bleed sometimes . I'm seeing a skin specialist about them.
What would happen if you did not wash your hands	I know deep down that nothing terrible would actually happen, I just that I get so wound up about it that I don't have a choice.
Family history of psychiatry illness	There's no one in my family who's mentally ill.
Personal history of psychiatric illness	I've never had any other psychiatric illnesses or medical illnesses. I've just always been anxious.
Drugs	I don't smoke or take drugs.

| *Hearing voices* | I don't hear any voices. I just wash my hands because I think they're dirty. |

| *Mood* | I'm not happy about that my cleanliness obsession is taking over my life, but I'm not down. |

Marking Scheme

2 marks: Good - 1 mark: Adequate - 0 mark: Poor/Not done	Mark 0 – 2
1. Polite introduction. Takes the patient's name.	☐
2. Finds extent of daily hand-washing.	☐
3. Finds duration of symptoms.	☐
4. Asks about cleaning routines.	☐
5. Finds out about obsessions	☐
6. Finds out about skin disorder.	☐
7. Finds out about its effects on her life.	☐
8. Asks about family history.	☐
9. Asks about medical history.	☐
10. Asks about previous psychiatric history.	☐
11. Excludes history of drug use.	☐
12. Excludes psychotic symptoms.	☐
13. Excludes depressive symptoms.	☐
14. Thanks the patient, overall impression.	☐

Examiner's additional questions (near the end)

Q: What is your diagnosis?	
15. A: Obsessive compulsive disorder.	☐

| TOTAL SCORE | / 30 |

Further information

Obsessive compulsive disorder (OCD) is defined by ICD-10 as obsessions or compulsions present on most days for at least 2 weeks and causing significant distress or interference with the patient's functioning. To reach this diagnosis, organic, drug-induced, psychotic and affective conditions must be excluded.

Obsessions are unwanted intrusive thoughts, images or urges (e.g. about contamination, order and symmetry, sex or violence), which in OCD are recognised as originating in the person's mind, so insight is maintained.

Compulsions are repetitive behaviours or mental acts which arise from obsessions, (e.g. washing, touch avoidance, checking, mantras, prayers), temporarily reducing anxiety, thus reinforcing themselves. OCD is listed by the WHO amongst the 10 most debilitating illnesses, in terms of lost income and decreased quality of life.

Drug treatment includes the selective serotonin reuptake inhibitors fluvoxamine and fluoxetine and the tricyclic clomipramine at high doses. However, response to these drugs can take up to 6 weeks and is required for up to 6 months, then tapered gradually.

Behaviour therapy techniques include response prevention, targeting rituals and avoidance behaviour.

OSCE 2 – History

Actor instructions
You are willing to talk about your problems but feel ashamed. You reveal more unprompted information when asked open questions and not interrupted.

When asked about	You mention
Your name	Hello I'm William Banks
Substance abuse	I've been drinking since I was fifteen, but more seriously in the last 3 years. During this time, I broke up with my fiancé. My family and my current girlfriend keep nagging me to cut down. At work, we go to a pub for lunch and have drinks every Friday. I go drinking with my mates on the weekend.
Drinking	I tend to drink about 4 pints of a Friday night and 6 shots. I drink about the same on a Saturday and 2 pints each lunch-time in the week. I don't tend to drink at home. I used to be more athletic but now have a beer belly.
Withdrawals	I don't get the shakes or any other symptoms when I stop drinking for a day or so. In the last 3 years, the longest I have gone without drink is one week. I tend to feel on edge approaching lunchtime, until I get my first drink. A few times I have drunk so much that I could not remember the previous night but never blacked out. I have never had jaundice, vomited blood or been admitted to hospital because of drinking. I don't drink and drive and have never had a drink-related injury.
Other substances	I smoke 10 cigarettes per day and occasionally take cocaine.
How often you take cocaine	I use it about once a month, only when I am drunk and spend about £30.

How you take co-caine (e.g injected? smoked?)	I snort cocaine, have never injected any drug or smoked anything other than cigarettes.
Effect on work	I am well known for my drinking at work, and more recently my boss has given me an official warning, and I'm "really scared".
Drunken incidents	While drunk and on coke last week I had an argument with my girlfriend and a mate. I threatened to punch my girlfriend in the mouth and grabbed my friend by his throat. When sober I apologised to them both and I feel ashamed. They didn't report it to the police and I have never been that violent before.
Self-harm	I have not thought about harming myself.
Family history	No one in my family is addicted to drugs or alcohol as far as I know.
How you feel	I think I have a drink problem and would like to cut down because it's upsetting my friends, affecting my health and costing too much money.

Marking Scheme	
2 marks: Good - 1 mark: Adequate - 0 mark: Poor/Not done	**Mark 0 – 2**
1. Introduces him/herself to patient.	
2. Explains that information is completely confidential.	
3. Elicits duration of heavy drinking.	
4. Elicits compulsive symptoms.	
5. Elicits weekly alcohol intake (48 units).	
6. Asks about withdrawal symptoms.	
7. Finds how substance use is affecting the rest of his life.	
8. Asks how he feels about his substance use.	
9. Finds out about drunken incidents and police involvement.	
10. Asks about ill-health caused by drinking, including accidents.	

11. Asks about other drug use. ☐
12. Asks about extent of other drug use and if he has injected. ☐
13. Asks about self-harm. ☐
14. Asks about family history of substance abuse. ☐
15. Thanks the patient, Overall impression. ☐

TOTAL SCORE **/ 30**

Further information
A unit is 8g or 10ml of ethanol, found in a half pint of beer, a glass (150ml) of wine or a shot (25ml) of spirits. The maximum safe daily limit is 4 units for men and 3 units for women, with maximum weekly limits of 21 and 14 units respectively.

Pregnant women or those trying for a baby are advised not to drink alcohol due to the risk of fetal alcohol syndrome, particularly in the first trimester. Average weekly consumption for UK men is 16 units, and for women 7 units (Office for National Statistics 2006).

A heavy drinker is classed as drinking twice the safe limit, but recall of amounts drunk is often underestimated. A binge is classed as >8 units in a day for a man or >6 units for a woman.

The **CAGE** questionnaire (Ever tried to **C**ut down? Are you **A**nnoyed when people tell you to? Ever feel **G**uilty about drinking? Do you ever have an **E**ye-cap (drink on waking)?) is good for screening but in this OSCE, you know the patient may have an addiction, not necessarily to alcohol. It is worth assessing him by the ICD-10 criteria.

Substance dependence ICD-10 criteria
(3+ for diagnosis, not necessarily simultaneous, over period of one year)

1. Strong compulsion to use substance
2. Difficulty controlling substance-taking behaviour
3. Withdrawal symptoms/ continuing use to avoid withdrawal
4. Signs of tolerance
5. Neglect of other activities
6. Continued use, despite awareness of damaging effects

This can be remembered using the mnemonic **SmACKHeaDS**- **S**trong compulsion to use, other **A**ctivities neglected, **C**ontinuing use to avoid withdrawal/ onset of withdrawal symptoms, continuing use despite **K**nowledge of **H**arm, **D**ifficulty controlling substance-taking behaviour, **S**igns of tolerance.

Alcohol abuse increases predisposition to subdural haemorrhage and affects many other systems. Alcoholic liver disease may be suggested by leuconychia (white nails), jaundice, nail clubbing, bruising, peripheral oedema (low albumin), hepatosplenomegaly, jaundice, , spider naevi, caput medusae, loss of body hair and ascites (fluid in peritoneal cavity).

Look also for sweating (during withdrawal), tremor, cerebellar signs and features of other drug use, such as injection marks, inflamed skin around the nose (glue-sniffing), pupil dilatation (cocaine, amphetamines) or constriction (opiates). Investigations relevant to substance abuse include FBC (macrocytic anaemia with alcohol abuse), LFT (ALT, AST, gamma GT elevated with alcohol abuse), HIV, Hepatitis B, C and D antibody tests, serum and urine drug levels. Liver imaging with ultrasound or CT may be required, with biopsy to investigate extent of disease.

To quantify health risks, it is important to know what drugs are being used and how they are administered. Injection can produce stronger effects from smaller amounts of drugs (may be started due to increasing tolerance and financial pressures), with attendant risks of infectious endocarditis, HIV and hepatitis.

If addicts are motivated, home detoxification, inpatient rehabilitation, group therapy and cognitive behavioural therapy are options, though facilities are often oversubscribed. Chlordiazepoxide and thiamine (vitamin B1), given intravenously in high-risk patients, can prevent alcohol withdrawal symptoms and Wernicke-Korsakoff syndrome.

OSCE 3 – History

Actor instructions
You appear fidgety and uncomfortable, sometimes hesitant in speech.
You reveal more unprompted information when asked open questions and not interrupted.

When asked about	You mention
Your name	My name is Jean Howie. I have been feeling nervy and on-edge for some time now.
How it started	I've noticed it more since my children were born. And it's been getting worse at work over the last year because they keep saying they will be making people redundant. My son is 10, my daughter is 7. I had heard about Down syndrome in older mums and was really worried in case they had it, but they are okay, touch wood. I've got this habit of calling their school from work just to check on them. They know who I am in the school office and my daughter gets embarrassed. They've got mobiles now and sometimes. I call to check on them at lunchtime. I know it's silly to keep calling but I just can't help myself, I imagine there's been an accident, you hear about all sorts of things happening. Sometimes this keeps me awake at night.
How it feels	My husband says I'm jumpy. When I get nervy about something, I can feel my heart beating faster, and I'm just sitting down. My hands start sweating, then they start shaking, and I feel like I have to run away or just crawl up into a ball. I get butterflies and can feel a bit sick. My palms would sweat and I'd be really embarrassed. I think my husband blames me for this, but it's not my fault, right? He's the one that told me to come here.

Voices or hallucinations	I have never "heard voices" or had hallucinations.
Mood/depression	My mood has not been low. I don't feel depressed. I work and look after my kids and am always busy.
Past medical history	I have never had any serious medical condition.
Drug history	I am not on any medication at the moment. I find that in social situations, gin can help my shakes.
Recreational drug use	I have never used drugs. I drink less than once a week.
Family history	I think I might be at risk of heart attack because my uncle had a heart attack. He was 70. My parents are in their seventies and reasonably healthy for their age.
If you have any questions	What do you think is causing my shakes?

Marking Scheme

2 marks: Good - 1 mark: Adequate - 0 mark: Poor/Not done — Mark 0 – 2

1. Polite introduction; verifies identity.
2. Finds duration of symptoms and situations that make her feel this way- i.e. everyday worries
3. Finds physical symptoms of anxiety
4. Excludes signs suggestive of psychosis.
5. Excludes signs suggestive of depression
6. Asks about past medical history
7. Asks for family history
8. Asks about drug history

9. Asks about alcohol/ recreational drug use (self-medication) ☐
10. Asks the patient if they have anything more to add/ any questions to ask ☐
11. Gives a satisfactory explanation of physical symptoms e.g. bio-feedback model ☐
12. Thanks the patient, Overall impression. ☐

Examiner's additional questions (near the end)

Q: What is the most likely diagnosis?
13. **A:** Generalised anxiety disorder. ☐

Q: What is the treatment?
14. **A:** Gives correct basic explanation of pharmacological and non-pharmacological treatment (see below). ☐

TOTAL SCORE / 28

Further information
To make a diagnosis of anxiety, conditions higher in the ICD-10 hierarchy like organic illness, drug effects, psychosis or a mood disorder that could cause the same symptoms, should be excluded. Generalised anxiety disorder is common, with a lifetime prevalence of ~12-17% and higher rates in females. The bio-feedback model refers to "fight or flight" adaptations during anxiety, which the patient notices, making them feel more anxious, causing more symptoms.

Cognitive behavioural therapy is a proven non-pharmacological intervention for generalised anxiety disorder, in which the patient is taught to understand the thinking behind their anxiety and develop more helpful ways of responding to stressful situations. Other treatments include SSRI's (e.g. paroxetine) and tricyclic antidepressants, particularly those with serotonergic effects like clomipramine. In the early stages, antidepressants may increase anxiety symptoms and need to be taken for at least 4 weeks before their effects start. If effective, treatment has to be maintained for a minimum of 6 months after optimal dose is reached, with weaning at the end to avoid withdrawal. Stopping treatment sooner than this may cause rebound anxiety/depression. Benzodiazepines may be used in the short-term (they work instantly), with weaning before 4 weeks, but they can cause rebound anxiety and dependency.

OSCE 4 – Explaining ECT

Actor instructions

You appear unhappy and only speak, slowly and quietly, when you are asked questions. You may need extra explanation but after asking questions you can give your valid consent to the procedure.

Examiner has a leaflet on ECT which they hand over if it is mentioned.

When asked	You mention
Your name	I'm Janine Adams.
How you feel	My mood has been low for 8 months. Depression has put the brakes on. I lost my job and fell behind payments on my flat. I live in a hostel now. I don't see my children. I feel tired all the time. I have no enjoyment in life.
If you have ever self-harmed	Last week I tried to commit suicide by overdosing. My mother happened to come round that night and she called the ambulance. I wish I hadn't done it now.
If you have had a recent brain haemorrhage, recent CVA, MI or arrhythmias	I have never had any of those.
About allergies	I have no allergies.
About your experience with general anaesthesia	I've never had an operation before.
If you have any questions	So I'll be awake?
To explain ECT (first time)	What happens again?

To explain ECT (second time)	Under general anaesthetic, I'll be shocked on one side of my head 6 times over 3 weeks.
To explain the purpose of ECT	This may help lift my depression.
To explain the risks of treatment	There is a risk of arrhythmias and agitation on regaining consciousness.
How you feel about treatment	I want to get better; I am willing to go ahead with this.

Marking Scheme

2 marks: Good - 1 mark: Adequate - 0 mark: Poor/Not done — Mark 0 – 2

1. Polite introduction, verifies identity.
2. Explains what they will do, asks permission.
3. Takes brief history of severe depression.
4. Takes history of suicide attempt, including current feelings.
5. Explains ECT procedure and purpose.
6. Explains risks of ECT.
7. Asks about contraindications.
8. Asks about allergies.
9. Asks about previous experience of anaesthesia.
10. Explains risks of not providing ECT.
11. Checks understanding: ▪ Asks to explain purpose
12. ▪ Asks to explain risks
13. Offers a leaflet on ECT (examiner provides it on mention).
14. Asks if they have any questions.
15. Takes consent on treatment in non-coercive fashion, tells the patient they can withdraw consent at any point.
16. Thanks the patient.

Examiner's additional questions (near the end)

Q: Is Ms Adam's consent valid?
17. **A:** The consent is valid.

> **Q: Why is it valid?**
> 18. **A:** She understands what the procedure entails, its potential risks and benefits and has not been coerced. ☐

TOTAL SCORE **/ 36**

Further information

Valid consent can be verbal or written and requires a non-coercive explanation that ensures the patient understands the procedure and the risks involved. Open questions (e.g. "How do you feel about it?", "What do you want me to explain again?") are better than yes/no directive and potentially coercive ones (e.g. "Is there anything you don't understand?" "Do you want to go ahead?"). Illness has to be severe and unresponsive to less radical therapies for ECT to be justified, with indications including severe depression, catatonic schizophrenia and prolonged or severe manic episodes. ECT requires section 58, with valid consent or the approval of a 2nd appointee, though in practice it is seldom done without the latter. In rare life-threatening psychiatric emergencies (e.g. stuporific patient refusing to drink), ECT can be given without consent or a second opinion. Bilateral ECT is more likely to cause amnesia.

The competent patient is defined as able to understand and retain information about the treatment, weigh its pros and cons and communicate their wishes. The Mental Capacity Act (2005) stipulates that doctors do their utmost to give patients the opportunity to demonstrate competence (e.g. provide translators, interview when they are most coherent). The Act created the role of Independent Mental Capacity Advocates, who liaise with the medical team in the interests of vulnerable patients unable to consent and without family or friends. No one can give consent on behalf of an incompetent adult; their treatment is based on the medical team's assessment of their best interests. Temporarily incapacitated patients can be treated under common law according to their best interests. Competent adults have the right to refuse life-saving treatment and any treatment forced on them may constitute battery.

OSCE 5 – History

Actor instructions
You are friendly and talk rapidly. Your words build a momentum, and you don't like being interrupted, but the student must do this occasionally to get the relevant information.

When asked about	You mention
Your name	Hello good day, my name is Vikesh Kambli. Nice to meet you, nice to meet you, welcome.
Presenting complaint	I don't think I have a problem. I'll say that again because I think it's of utmost importance. I don't think I have a problem. My lovely wife asked me to come here. My loyal GP asked me to come here.
	I am a very successful businessman. I wear princely clothes. If I see a coat I like, I buy that coat. I put it on the plastic. Credit card not a debit card. No problem. I'm not in the red.
	There are God people and devil people. There are spiritual people and there are non-spiritual people. Any question you ask me I will look you in the eye and tell you the truth as I see it. God sees everything. Whether you pray to Krishna, you pray to Allah you pray to Jehovah, there is only one God and God is great. All God's people are my people. Do you understand? I'm a spiritual person. If I see shoes for my wife, I buy shoes for my wife, no problem.
Duration of symptoms	They could have been telling me that for 2 months they could have been telling me that for 5 months. I have 2 children. 2 sons. If you can't give your children a moral grounding you can't give them anything. My parents passed on to me that you can't get anything unless you work for it. Listen, I built a business from nothing, from a thousand pound loan and now it joyously bears

211

fruit. The trees have got no leaves this time of year. My wife's talking to me about a separation, but I don't want a separation, you understand me? I have one wife and one wife alone, but if I wanted I could find another in 2 days. I tell my sons I love them. I take them aside and tell them this specifically with a pat on the head and a handshake. My wife takes me aside and she says she loves me. My friends take me aside and say that they love me. My sons take me aside and say that they love me. If you come near my house, I will cook you a meal, beautiful food. Women stare at me on buses, in trains. I ask them to marry me, they would say yes. And now we import from three continents. My wife can't take that away, my brother can't take that away, my GP can't take that away.

Sleep habits

Sleep, I don't need to sleep. 2 or 3 hours maximum. Why sleep when I've got a business to run, my wife to take care of, my children to take care of? Time is the enemy, that's what Napoleon said. You give me your business and I can make it as successful as my own. I've got to the top, you understand? People ask me "Vikesh, how do you do it?" Tell me how you run things, I'll tell you how I run things and you can do the same as me. One day I want to write book about how to make business successful. One day I want to have my own television show on how to make businesses. But now I give it all away for free.

About general health

I've never been ill a day in my life, not one day. I worked hard for my family. I work hard for my own self-esteem. Family is the most important thing.

If hearing voices

Well I'm hearing your voice, buster. But I don't hear other voices. I don't need to hear voices. I think for myself. I speak for myself. I could be a voice for those people. If I got the time to do that,

I could do a lot of good that way, a lot of good. I would only listen to God people and I would say what God people wanted me to say and they would revere me for that. People get intimidated in the spotlight, but I don't get intimidated in the spotlight. I can go in the community I can talk to the community I can find what the problems are. I can talk to you on a level, I can talk to high people I can talk to low people. I carry a message I get it across. Telecommunications are very powerful but what if the email machine breaks down? What if the telephone breaks down? Don't build your house on sand. Build your house with solid foundations and you will go very far.

Beliefs or special powers

My special power is the love of my family. My belief is a belief in God and the human race. Thanks.

Mood

I have never been depressed on day in my life. That's just how I am. Depression is one of the great obstacles in this country. Winston Churchill was depressed, Elvis Presley was depressed. If I was depressed I would lose my drive.

Medication

I'm not on medication, I don't need medication, I'm not ill. Ill people need medication. Side-effects are unintended and can be highly dangerous.

Recreational drugs

I don't do drugs. I'm clean. Young people do drugs because they have too much pocket money. I'm not young and I don't have pocket money, therefore I do not do drugs.

Family history

My mother is healthy, my father is healthy. My son Rahul is healthy, my son Ramu is healthy. My wife Preethi is healthy. How is your family?

If you have any questions

I don't have any questions. I enjoy talk to intelligent people. I enjoy talk to goodhearted people.

Marking Scheme	
2 marks: Good - 1 mark: Adequate - 0 mark: Poor/Not done	**Mark 0 – 2**

1.	Polite introduction, verifies identity.	☐
2.	Finds duration of episode.	☐
	Elicits manic features:	
3.	▪ Grandiosity (belief in extraordinary business acumen, attractiveness etc)	☐
4.	▪ Increased pleasurable activity without thought of consequences (i.e. spending sprees)	☐
5.	▪ Increased talkativeness	☐
6.	▪ Decreased need for sleep	☐
7.	▪ Flight of ideas (jumps between loosely-linked subjects, rhyme/ clang associations)	☐
8.	▪ Increased goal-driven activity	☐
9.	Enquires about mood previously.	☐
10.	Enquires about drug history.	☐
11.	Enquires about recreational drug use.	☐
	Enquires about psychotic features:	
12.	▪ Hallucinations	☐
13.	▪ Special powers/other delusions	☐
14.	Enquires about past medical history.	☐
15.	Enquires about past psychiatric history.	☐
16.	Asks about family history.	☐
17.	Asks if the patient has any questions.	☐
18.	Thanks the patient.	☐

Examiner's additional questions (near the end)	
Q: What is the diagnosis?	
19. A: Bipolar disorder, manic phase without psychosis.	☐
Q: What treatment is available?	
20. A: Gives correct basic explanation of treatment e.g. initial atypical antipsychotic treatment combined with lithium.	☐

TOTAL SCORE	**/ 40**

Further information

As Mr Kambli has pressure of speech, the student has to know when to interrupt him to ask key questions and when to hold back, for example when his monologue discloses his grandiosity, flight of ideas, increased activity and spending sprees. Though he isn't psychotic, he is grandiose, with impaired insight and an inflated view of his place in the world.

Mania can cause mood-congruent psychosis in the form of secondary delusions. Mania without psychosis is a disorder defined by ICD-10 as elevated, expansive or irritable mood, abnormal for the individual and disruptive of everyday life, comprising 3 or more of the following features (4 if the mood is irritable not elated) over a period of at least 1 week:

- Inflated self-esteem or grandiosity.
- Behaviour which is foolhardy or reckless and whose risks the subject doesn't recognize e.g. spending sprees.
- Increased activity or physical restlessness.
- Distractibility or constant changes in activity or plans.
- Loss of normal social inhibitions resulting in behaviour which is inappropriate to the circumstances.
- Decreased need for sleep.
- Marked sexual energy or sexual indiscretions.
- Flight of ideas or the experience of thoughts racing.
- Increased talkativeness ('pressure of speech').

These can be remembered using the mnemonic **GRAnDIoSITy**- **G**randiosity or inflated self-esteem, **R**eckless behavior, increased **A**ctivity, **D**istractibility and **D**isinhibition, **I**nsomnia, marked **S**exual energy, flight of **I**deas, increased **T**alkativeness.

Other features of mania include self-neglect, aggression plus heightened colour and sound perception. Hypomania is less severe and lasts less than a week. Cyclothymia is mood instability that doesn't fit the criteria of hypomania, mania or depression. Bipolar affective disorder can be classed as bipolar I (depression and mania), bipolar II (depression and hypomania) Depressive phases last ~6 months, with manic phases shorter and becoming less often with age. Psychosis is common with mania, but is mood congruent e.g. a fixed, false and culturally inappropriate belief of controlling the stock market or hallucinating complimentary voices. Organic diseases that can cause manic symptoms include frontal CVA, multiple sclerosis and systemic lupus erythematosus, as can the use of stimulant drugs. Mania presenting for the first time in adults over 65 is more strongly associated with organic causes (Tohen et al 1994).

	Manic features	Schizophrenic features
Thought form	Thought flight	Loosening of association, alogia, neologisms
Delusions	Mood-congruent	Bizarre, delusions of thought, delusions of passivity, delusions of perception
Speech	Increased amount, pressured	May be reduced
Biological	Reduced sleep, increased energy, self-neglect	Self neglect
Psychomotor	Agitation	Agitation, catatonia (rare), flat/ incongruent affect

OSCE 6 – History

Actor instructions

You are willing to talk, looking for answers and acknowledgement. You reveal more unprompted information when the student asks open questions and doesn't interrupt. One minute from the end, you ask the student what is causing your symptoms. You take offence at insinuations of mental illness, or it being "all in the mind."

When asked about	You mention
Your name	Hello my name is Marie Jenkins.
Presenting complaint	I have not been feeling well for some time now. I have had back problems on and off for 7 years. In recent months I've been feeling tired all the time. This isn't like me because I am a very active person normally. I find it difficult to get to sleep and get fluttering chest pains sometimes. I get headaches too, like a drilling pain around my temples and burning in my stomach. Afternoons, especially, I can feel really bloated, I'm intolerant of apples. I'm always getting coughs and colds, whenever they're going round I get them. I'm always thinking about what is bringing on these problems, do you think it could be my immune system?
Past medical history	I had a really serious urine tract infection last year. The doctor gave me trimethoprim, which gave me terrible diarrhoea. Three years ago I had an operation for carpal tunnel syndrome, and I have been investigated for loads of diseases.
Previous investigations	Last time I went to A & E, they gave me a chest x-ray, they said it was clear. I was referred for an ECG last year, which at the time they said was normal. Earlier this year I had a camera down my throat to look at my stomach. Though I was having symptoms just like an ulcer, they said it wasn't. A few years ago I had an MRI of my back which they said was normal.

Drug history	I'm not on anything. Just the oral contraceptive pill and occasionally aspirin.
Recreational drugs	No, I would never ever do that.
Family history	My parents are both alive and in their sixties. My father has angina but is otherwise well. I have a sister and had a brother, who died fifteen years ago when he crashed his car. My sister had bulimia when she was a teenager, but she's fine now. I have 3 very energetic and healthy sons aged 7, 6 and 4.
Hearing voices	I don't hear voices or anything like that.
Mood	I don't feel so bad. I have friends that are depressed and that used to be depressed and I don't feel like that. I've not been losing weight or anything like that.
What you think is causing the symptoms	I don't know. It just seems like one thing after another sometimes, my oldest son is getting in trouble at school plus I'm not getting on with my husband. I just feel really stressed.
How your symptom have affected your life	My husband works as a baker but recently he has been worried about his income. Before my children were born, I worked in admin. I have been meaning to go back for some time as all my children are in school, but I've not been feeling that well. Me and my husband have had a few arguments about my health problems. It just makes them worse. Sometimes I'm so tired I don't pick my kids up from school on time and he gets really angry. I don't mean to be like this.
Why you have presented now	I have seen the GP several times. Things are getting more stressful at home. I want to find out what's wrong and what I can do about it. Things are coming to a head at home and my husband doesn't like me complaining.

What you would like to be done	I'd just like to get to the bottom of this. I want to get on with my life, get a job, work, whatever. What do you think is causing all this?

Marking Scheme

2 marks: Good - 1 mark: Adequate - 0 mark: Poor/Not done	Mark 0 – 2
1. Polite introduction, verifies identity.	☐
2. Asks about past medical history and treatment.	☐
3. Asks about drug history.	☐
4. Asks about recreational drug use.	☐
5. Asks about family history.	☐
6. Finds out about previous investigations.	☐
7. Excludes psychosis.	☐
Excludes affective disorder:	
8. ▪ Asks about mood level	☐
9. ▪ Asks about other biological symptoms of depression	☐
10. Asks patient what she thinks is the cause.	☐
11. Asks how symptoms have affected the patient's life.	☐
12. Asks what she would like/ if she has any questions.	☐
13. Explains provisional diagnosis of **somatization** in a diplomatic way, linking stress to physical manifestations.	☐
14. Thanks the patient. Overall impression.	☐

Examiner's additional questions (near the end)

Q: What is your provisional diagnosis?	
15. **A:** Suspected somatization disorder.	☐
Q: How would you find out more about her symptoms?	
16. **A:** Examine her and obtain further information e.g. interviewing her family, reviewing her notes, discussion with multidisciplinary team, avoiding unnecessary investigations.	☐

TOTAL SCORE	/ 32

Further information
Somatization, classed amongst the somatoform disorders, is the expression of psychological distress as medically unexplained symptoms; organic, drug-related, psychotic and mood disorders must be excluded before it is diagnosed. Somatization typically features symptoms from several systems, with typical complaints including back pain, dysuria, bloating, colicky abdominal pain, non-ulcer dyspepsia, palpitations, tension, headaches, tiredness and insomnia. It is important to clinically assess each complaint seriously in order to evaluate the risk of organic disease. Red flags of organic disease, such as a history of treated cancer (even following an "all clear"), should push somatization down the list of differentials. Early metastatic disease may manifest as unexplained pain, with nothing detected on imaging.

The greater the number of unrelated complaints, which tend not to fit typical patterns of organic illness, the higher the likelihood that somatization may be involved. Somatization can cause dangerous investigations and treatments to be wrongly given, while overlooking genuine organic illness, which may occur alongside somatization symptoms, is also perilous.

Complying with requests for unnecessary investigations and specialist referrals may further convince patients of physical illness, while an accusatory approach is also unhelpful. The "re-attribution" model requires an empathic exploration of their health problems and social issues, by which their discomfort is acknowledged and re-attributed to stressful life events.

The doctors seeing the patient should agree who has primary responsibility and organise regular brief appointments, avoiding repeated reassurance as this encourages dependency. The goal should be a graded return to previous activity levels.

OSCE 7 – Written station

1.

$40kg/ (64 \times 0.0254m)^2 = 15.14kg/m^2$

2.

The 4 ICD-10 defining features of anorexia nervosa are:

- Body mass index less than $17.5kg/m^2$ or less than 85% expected weight.
- Endocrine disturbance e.g. amenorrhoea lasting 3+ cycles (when not on the pill), hypothyroidism, delayed puberty.
- Overvalued idea leading to a dread of obesity and a feeling they are overweight.
- Deliberate weight loss e.g. by dieting and exercise, vomiting, use of medication.

 These may be remembered using the mnemonic **WElgheD** i.e. reduced **W**eight, **E**ndocrine disturbance, overvalued **I**dea, **D**eliberate weight loss.

Other clinical features may include:

- **Cardiovascular**: hypotension, bradycardia, arrhythmias from electrolyte imbalance, peripheral oedema (hypoalbuminaemia).
- **Gastrointestinal**: emaciation, constipation, abdominal pain, diarrhoea (from laxative abuse), hepatomegaly, ascites, leuconychia, repeated vomiting causing tooth decay, callused hand (Russell's sign), and swollen salivary glands.
- **Neurological/ Psychological**: proximal myopathy, lethargy, depression.
- **Endocrine**: amenorrhoea, reproductive system atrophy, lanugo, cold intolerance, hair loss.

3.

Female (~10 females: 1male), living in North America or Western Europe, high social class background, being from white racial background, family history, high-risk occupations: model, ballerina.

4.

FBC, TFT, U&E, LFT, serum FSH/LH, vitamin B12, calcium, phosphate, folate, ferritin, total iron binding capacity and magnesium levels.

5.

- **Endocrine**: hypothyroidism, amenorrhoea, impotence, delayed puberty, growth retardation.
- **Cardiovascular**: anaemia, heart failure
- **Gastrointestinal**: hypoglycaemia, oesophageal tear, gastric rupture, electrolyte imbalances e.g. hypokalaemia, hypochloraemic alkalosis from vomiting.
- **Neurological**: weakness, seizures.
- **Other**: osteoporosis, increased risk of infection.

6.

Psychological approaches like group therapy and cognitive behavioural therapy target the overvalued idea, together with medical treatment to deal with its physical complications, aiming for a steady gain of 1.5 kg per week, with final BMI 20-25. Antidepressants may be used for co-morbid depression or obsessive compulsive disorder.

Further information

Anorexia nervosa is classed as a behavioural disorder in the ICD-10 diagnostic hierarchy, to be considered after organic, drug-related, psychotic, affective and anxiety-related conditions have been excluded. Incidence is ~20 per 100 000 women per year in the UK (~10 times less common in men). ~40% of people make a full recovery, ~30% have fluctuating illness and mortality is ~10%, by suicide or medical complications. Poor prognostic factors include associated bulimia, extreme weight loss, late onset, long duration and poor family support. As anorexia nervosa and bulimia nervosa are much rarer in less economically developed countries, they are considered by some to be culturally-specific disorders.

OSCE 8 – Clozapine treatment

Actor instructions
You appear calm and reasonable, though not talkative. If the candidate uses jargon, you ask for an explanation.

Examiner has a leaflet about clozapine for the patient that is kept concealed until the candidate mentions it.

When asked about	You mention
Your name	I'm John Ferris.
Psychiatric history	This all started a year ago, I'm 28 now. The worst was going round streets at night, thinking people were about to attack me. Even at the running club, I'd think I could hear them talking bad things, even with the medication. My life's on the pause button. My CV's got a hole in the middle. So the situation at the moment is pretty serious.
Drug history	They started me on risperidone. That had a bit of an effect, but I'd still be getting para. That lasted 3 months, then they tried me on olanzapine, for 6 weeks and that didn't work so well either, I could still hear the voices.
Other medication and drugs	I don't take any other medication and I have never done drugs.
Adherence	I always took them when they said. The pack comes with times on it, next to every pill, so you know if you miss them anyway.
Past medical history	I've never had any blood disease, heart disease, epilepsy. I've not got diabetes.
If you have any questions	What are the other options?
How you feel starting on clozapine	I'll battle on, try and achieve something. I trust my psychiatrist's judgement.

Marking Scheme	
2 marks: Good - 1 mark: Adequate - 0 mark: Poor/Not done	**Mark 0 – 2**
1. Polite introduction, verifies identity.	☐
2. Takes brief history of psychiatric symptoms.	☐
3. Takes drug history- i.e. checks clozapine is really indicated.	☐
4. Asks about drug adherence.	☐
5. Asks about other drug use.	☐
6. Asks about relevant cautionary and contraindicating conditions.	☐
7. Explains indications for clozapine use.	☐
8. Explains side effects of clozapine.	☐
9. Explains importance of reporting signs of infection.	☐
10. Explains role of monitoring commission and the investigations required before he can start treatment.	☐
11. Asks for questions.	☐
12. Provides reasonable alternative options e.g. other atypical and typical antipsychotics are possible options, but clozapine is recommended in his case.	☐
13. Asks the patient how he feels about starting clozapine.	☐
14. Asks the patient to take a leaflet (at which point examiner hands it over).	☐
15. Overall impression.	☐
TOTAL SCORE	**/ 30**

Further information

Clozapine should be initiated when other antipsychotic drugs have been tapered off. In drug-resistant schizophrenia, clozapine can be expected to control symptoms in 30-50% of cases, perhaps rising to 60% over 12 months.

OSCE 9 – Explaining autism

Actor instructions

You don't know much about autism but are willing to listen. You speak more about your son's history when asked open questions and not interrupted.

Examiner has a leaflet on autism for the patient that is kept concealed until the candidate mentions it.

When asked about	You mention
Your name	Hello, my name is Gina Desmond.
Your current understanding	I recently found out my son Jeffrey has autism. I don't know much about it.
Your son's development	He is 6, but we worried about him from before this. He was late to start talking, he said his first word when he was 5. Now he has perhaps 10 words he uses regularly and he can say only very basic sentences.
	As a baby, he was late smiling, at least compared to our other son Mark. Jack plays alone, but can get really angry if Mark interrupts him.
	He spends ages obsessing about his cars being in line, but doesn't play with them so much, just sets them as arrangements.
If you have any questions	▪ Jack had his 2 MMR vaccinations, could this have caused the autism? ▪ What has caused the autism? ▪ What is the treatment? ▪ If I had another child, what would the risk be of he or she having autism?

Marking Scheme	
2 marks: Good - 1 mark: Adequate - 0 mark: Poor/Not done	**Mark 0 – 2**

1. Polite introduction. Verifies identity. ☐
2. Asks what they understand about autism. ☐
3. Takes brief history of son's development. ☐

Explains 3 features of autism
4. ▪ Late speech development ☐
5. ▪ Strong tendency to avoid social contact ☐
6. ▪ Stereotyped interests, behaviours or routines. ☐

7. Mentions support available: educational support, speech and language therapy, special schools, disability benefit, makaton communication aid, chat rooms etc ☐
8. Explains severity varies but gives realistic prognosis: risk of never being fully independent and learning disabilities. ☐
9. Majority develop useful speech. ☐
10. Mentions leaflet available/ National Autistic Society ☐
11. Asks for questions. ☐
12. Explains why MMR vaccination is safe (just because autistic features first emerge after MMR vaccination, it does not follow that they are caused by it. ☐
13. Explains cause is unknown in most cases, gives examples of causes such as congenital rubella, prematurity. ☐
14. Explains there is no treatment, but mentions examples of support such as self-help groups, social services ☐
15. Explains autism is rare, so the chances another child having autism are low. ☐

TOTAL SCORE | **/ 30**

Further information

Autism is a pervasive developmental disorder, idiopathic in most cases but causes include early brain damage (e.g. congenital rubella infection, prematurity, phenylketonuria). Prevalence estimates vary from 1 per 2500 to 1 per 100 (with ~3:1 male: female ratio), higher figures including a larger proportion without learning disabilities.

Makaton is a sign and symbol-based language programme for teaching literacy and language skills to people with communication difficulties. No medication is available for autism itself, but anticonvulsants may be required (~20% develop epilepsy).

Families of autistic people may benefit from social services input, self-help groups and assistance from the National Autistic Society.

A small study involving 12 subjects by Wakefield et al (1998), speculated upon a link between MMR vaccination (given at 12-15 months and 3-4 years) and autism, later refuted by most of its authors. Government reassurance couldn't prevent falling vaccination rates, leading in 2006 to the first UK measles fatality since 1992. Large retrospective cohort studies involving thousands of subjects in Denmark (Madsen et al 2005), and Japan (Honda et al 2005) found no increased incidence of autism in children vaccinated with MMR. The fact that autistic signs develop around the age of MMR vaccination and the increasing use of "autistic spectrum" as a diagnosis (meaning more children are included) both contributed to the spread of this medical myth.

The triple vaccine enables greater coverage, because fewer children would complete 6 separate doses. 95% immunization levels are required for "herd immunity". ~454 000 children died from measles in 2004, MMR is endorsed by the WHO (500 million doses given since 1972) and was created by Dr Maurice Hilleman (1919-2005); his measles vaccine alone saves ~1 million children's lives per year.

OSCE 10 – Mental test score

Actor instructions
Your name is Agnes Bellman. You are irritable but agree to do the mental test that the doctor is offering. You will be asked 10 questions by the doctor. Make sure that you answer exactly 3 questions wrong.

Marking Scheme	
2 marks: Good - 1 mark: Adequate - 0 mark: Poor/Not done	**Mark 0 – 2**
1. Polite introduction. Verifies identity.	☐
2. Explains what the test they are about to perform and asks permission.	
3. Asks for the patient's date of birth.	☐
4. Asks them to remember an address (e.g. 29 Canver street)	☐
5. Asks what time it is.	☐
6. Asks what day it is.	
7. Asks what month it is.	☐
8. Asks what year it is.	☐
9. Asks them where they are now.	☐
10. Asks for the dates of World War 2.	☐
11. Asks for the name of the Prime Minister.	☐
12. Asks to count backward from 20 to 1.	☐
13. Asks to repeat the address.	☐
Examiner's additional questions (near the end)	
Q: What was Mrs Bellman's score?	
14. **A:** Gives correct score of 7/10.	☐
Q: What does this score mean?	
15. **A:** Says 7/10 means a mild impairment of cognition.	☐
Q: What are some possible causes?	
16. **A:** Examples include dementia and acute confusional state, causes of which include acute infection and medication.	☐
TOTAL SCORE	**/ 32**

Further information

The abbreviated mental test is a brief test for assessing cognition. A score of 8 or more is classed normal, 4-7 mildly impaired, <4 moderate to severely impaired. Acute confusional state differs from dementia in that it involves a reduced level of consciousness and it can be brought on by seemingly unrelated insults like a urinary tract infection. The mini-mental state examination takes longer but is more detailed; test yourself on this over 10 minutes when you are confident at the 10-point test. Neuropsychometric testing is more detailed and may be performed to assess function following brain injuries.

Mini mental state examination

Orientation in time:
- Name the year, season, month, date and day (5 points).

Orientation in space:
- Name the country, region, town, building and ward you are in (5 points).

Attention:
- Subtract 7 from 100 and repeat 4 times, or spell "world" backwards (5 points).

Registration:
- Repeat back three words that the examiner says and remember them for later, said in a row (3 points).

Language:
- Name 2 objects or people that the examiner points out (2 points).
- Write a sentence (correct grammar not required) (1 point).
- Read aloud what is written on this piece of paper and do what it says ("close your eyes" is written) (1 point).
- Copy this design (presented with 2 overlapping pentagons) (1 point).
- Listen to the examiner and repeat what they say (no 'ifs', 'ands', or 'buts') (1 point).
- Conduct a 3-stage command as told to you by the examiner (e.g. "lift your right hand, point at the ceiling and touch your left knee", with no prompting, repetition or gestures from the examiner) (3 points).

Recall:
- Repeat back the 3 words given to you earlier (3 points).

Scores of 25-27 out of 30 are borderline. Less than 25 suggests dementia but can also be caused by depression or acute confusional state. A score between 10 and 20 suggests moderate dementia, while less than 10 suggests severe dementia.

OSCE 11 – Explaining schizophrenia

Actor instructions
You are keen to know about the disease. You react badly if bluntly told about 10% suicide risk. If the student uses too much jargon, you ask them to clarify.

Examiner has a leaflet on schizophrenia which is revealed when the candidate mentions it, otherwise it is concealed.

When asked about	You mention
Your name	My name is Lisa Rutherford.
Your current understanding	My brother has been having problems for the last few months. He reacts to voices that no one else can hear and gets frightened and angry for no reason. I don't know much about schizophrenia.
If you have any questions	• Is a psychopath the same as a schizophrenic? • Does this mean that I am more likely to become schizophrenic?

Marking Scheme	
2 marks: Good - 1 mark: Adequate - 0 mark: Poor/Not done	**Mark 0 – 2**
1. Polite introduction. Verifies identity.	☐
2. Asks about current understanding of illness.	☐
3. Explains schizophrenia is common: ~1% lifetime risk.	☐
Describes features of schizophrenia- e.g 4. • Auditory hallucination: perceiving voices originating in the mind as if from the surrounding environment.	☐
5. • Delusion: false and culturally inappropriate fixed belief e.g. that thoughts are being broadcast to others.	☐
6. Explains other features e.g. nonsensical speech, paranoia, inappropriate mood, illogical thinking, social withdrawal.	☐

7. Explains treatment- oral antipsychotics, possible depot ☐
   injection, likely to be long-term.
8. Explains treatment given in the community by mental health ☐
   team, section possible under the mental health act.
9. Explains prognosis in a sensitive manner. ☐
10. Explains prognostic factors with emphasis on those that can ☐
    be changed e.g. drug concordance, expressed emotion,
    avoidance of drug abuse.
11. Mentions leaflet or group e.g. MIND (whereupon examiner ☐
    hands it to actress)
12. Asks for questions. ☐
13. Explains schizophrenia causes "psychotic" features such ☐
    as hallucinations or delusions, while "psychopath" is some-
    thing else entirely, referring to someone with reduced ca-
    pacity for empathy and remorse and no difficulty judging
    what is real.
14. Explains family history is one of many risk factors and her ☐
    risk may be slightly higher. However, non-genetic
    factors such as birth trauma, drug use and life stresses may
    not apply to her.
15. Overall impression ☐

TOTAL SCORE | **/ 30**

Further information
Risk factors for schizophrenia include family history, living in inner-city areas, being a second generation Afro-Caribbean person in the UK (diagnostic bias may influence), poverty (according to environmental breeder hypothesis), birth trauma and being male (~1.4:1 bias).

Schizophrenia's lifetime prevalence is ~1% with incidence rates of 16-42 per 100 000 people per year (Jablensky, 2000). Positive symptoms are more likely during acute relapses, acute onset of disease and in younger patients. Negative symptoms tend to be chronic and are commoner in older patients, though mixtures of both can occur in the same person.

When most schizophrenic patients were locked away, they were prone to developing negative symptoms due to the lack of stimulation offered them. An excess of stimulation, through high expressed emotion of the patient's family, pleasant or unpleasant changes in their life can induce relapse with positive symptoms.

Positive prognostic factors in schizophrenia include being female, living with people of low expressed emotion, early diagnosis and treatment, having an acute onset in later life, good social support, a large affective component to disease, primarily positive symptoms and no family history of schizophrenia. ~80% of newly-diagnosed schizophrenic people will experience a relapse, ~25% will have 1-2 episodes then recover fully, ~50% will have chronic relapsing illness, ~25% will have poor outcome including ~10% who commit suicide.

Life expectancy in the UK is reduced by ~10 years, with more social stressors, higher smoking rates and consequent morbidities.

OSCE 12 – History

Actor instructions
You are suspicious, using neologisms. When asked sensitively, you talk of your symptoms openly, but are irritated by suggestions you are psychotic. You reveal more unprompted information when asked open questions and not interrupted.

When asked about	You mention
Your name	I'm John Randolph.

Presenting complaint

I've been imprisoned over 2 weeks. The f*****g CIA, MI5, Al Qaeda and Mossad have been harassing me for 3 months. I don't know what the shenjacks have planned. My room-mate is working for Mossad. The CIA monitors the UK. Israel invaded Egypt and Britain bloody helped them to do it. My roommate put a camera in the toilet that only I can see. He hasn't told me but I know it's there because of the piss marks he left on the floor. He's an undercover but he doesn't want to be an undercover because he likes me. He puts semen in my sandwiches but I don't eat semen sandwiches, you understand?

Past medical

I never had problems as a child. I was always a healthy child. I am at the apogee of health, I have never had any operations apart from when I was captured here and the CIA surgeons placed a microchip in my leg to monitor my thoughtsAnd if I concentrate hard enough, I can destroy it. The information they want lives in the brain behind my right eye. Once that's gone I'll be safe.

Substance abuse

I have taken cocaine in the past but I have not touched illegal substances for 2 years. I drink on the weekends sometimes enough to get drunk, but not always enough to get drunk, up to ten pints over 2 days. When I'm thirsty I drink. When I'm hungry I eat. The Chinese secret police is the worst secret police. It's not safe to be in college.

Hearing voices	I hear the robot voices monitoring me. Mossad want me to work for them. Al-Qaeda want me to work for them. The bloody CIA want me to work for them. I have all the talents. I don't want to work for anyone, I work for myself and for society, you understand? I don't believe in margonia. All violence is wrong. I'd be happy when I'm out of this dungeon. Just give me adequate security assurances, grant me that basic respect. They did it to Vanunu they will do it to me. Their secrets are dangerous secrets. It's got to the point I can't even have sex in case she's part of the act. I never want to become a gigolo for the CIA. Being in prison here, or being in prison in Israel or being in prison in Cuba, I'd choose here. But it costs a lot to keep me here. And if extremists got hold of my secrets, it would cost everyone. And that's not a threat, that's a scientific fact.
Control of your thoughts	Sometimes the microchip sends my thoughts out to the CIA supercomputer. It buzzes.
Control of your body	I am in full control of my actions. It is normal to be in full control of your actions.
Past psychiatric history	I have never been mentally ill.
Self-harm	Listen, I've got CIA agents outside my flat, I've got Mossad outside my flat. How would you feel about that? I was thinking of jumping in front of a train because at least that would end it, you know what I mean?
Social history	I live with my mother, my father and my brother. I used to study in college and work at a printing firm. The area where I live is a dangerous area. Don't joke, you can't go out at night.. There's myries in my area. Ask anyone, if you go out at night on my estate, the people are all on drugs and ready to rape you, rob you, kill you. You

can't dress like you dress on my estate. I've had bad experiences in the past and I've had good experiences in the past

Family history   My family is well.

Medication   They give me medication and I take medication.

Marking Scheme	
2 marks: Good - 1 mark: Adequate - 0 mark: Poor/Not done	**Mark 0 – 2**

1. Polite introduction. Verifies identity. ☐
2. Asks about past medical history. ☐
3. Asks about substance abuse. ☐
4. Elicits duration of strange behaviour. ☐
5. Elicits history of delusions of perception (urine means his roommate is an agent). ☐
6. Elicits history of bizarre delusions (he is wanted by several international organisations). ☐
7. Elicits history of thought delusions (withdrawal by computer chip). ☐
8. Asks about delusions of passivity (i.e. thoughts or actions are being controlled by others). ☐
9. Elicits history of hallucinations- third person auditory (robot voices), somatic hallucination (buzzing chip). ☐
10. Elicits paranoid feelings. ☐
11. Asks about past history of psychiatric illness. ☐
12. Asks about deliberate self-harm. ☐
13. Elicits drug history. ☐
14. Asks about social history. ☐
15. Asks about family history. ☐
16. Thanks the patient. Overall impression. ☐

Examiner's additional questions (near the end)

Q: What is the diagnosis?
17. **A:** Paranoid schizophrenia (1 mark for schizophrenia). ☐

TOTAL SCORE **/ 34**

Further information

	Symptoms in schizophrenia	
	Positive	**Negative**
Appearance	Elaborate headgear e.g. tinfoil (protective in regard to thought delusions), luminous clothing.	Lack of reward behaviour: weight loss, poor hygiene, lack of self-care.
Behaviour	Psychomotor agitation.	Psychomotor retardation, apathy, poor eye contact.
Speech	Incoherent with neologisms, loosening of association (jumping between apparently unrelated topics) e.g. word salad, clang and pun associations.	Poverty of speech.
Thought	Delusions.	Alogia (loss of logical thought).
Cognition	Reduced concentration. Orientation often normal.	Cognitive ability possibly reduced.
Mood	Agitation, incongruent affect (may smile about sad event).	Flattened affect- total lack of expressed emotion, anhedonia- loss of pleasurable activity.
Perceptions	Hallucinations with reactions e.g. talking, laughing with no one else around.	Hallucinations possible, though reactions may be minor.

There is much to elicit in just 5 minutes, he has florid psychotic features. Certain symptoms such as delusions of thought need to be asked about directly, for example "how have you been feeling about the control of your thoughts recently?"

Schizophrenia can only be diagnosed if organic and drug causes of the psychiatric symptoms are excluded. A diagnosis of schizophrenia is avoided if there are marked depressive or manic symptoms (suggesting manic or depressive psychosis), unless the schizophrenia predates them.

There are 4 subtypes of schizophrenia: paranoid (most common), hebephrenic (disorganized), catatonic or undifferentiated. If and affective components alternate at roughly equal intensity, the diagnosis is schizoaffective disorder.

<u>ICD-10 Basic Criteria for Schizophrenia</u> must have been present for at least one month and not due to organic disease or drug usage.

<u>Group 1</u> (only 1 required for diagnosis)
a. Delusions of thought insertion/ withdrawal/ broadcast
b. Delusions of control/passivity/ perception clearly referred to body or limb movements or specific thoughts, actions, sensations.
c. Hallucinatory voices in 1st or 3rd person.
d. Bizarre delusions- culturally inappropriate and impossible.

<u>Group 2</u> (2 required for diagnosis as these are less specific)
e. Persistent hallucination when accompanied by delusion without clear affective component
f. Neologisms, breaks, interpolations in train of thought and loosening of association leading to incoherent, irrelevant speech (word salad or verbigeration).
g. Catatonic features, which can manifest with hyperactive (purposeless or stereotyped movements, mannerisms, echolalia, echopraxia) or re-duced (posturing, mutism) motor activity.
h. Negative symptoms such as marked apathy, paucity of speech, pov-erty of thought, self-neglect, emotional blunting (not due to depression or medication)

Group 1 features can be remembered using the mnemonic **sCHIZ**- delusions of **C**ontrol/passivity, auditory **H**allucinations in 1st or 3rd person, thought **I**nsertion/ withdrawal/ broadcast, bi**Z**arre delu-sions.

Group 2 features can be remembered using the mnemonic **OPHreNIC**- **O**ther **P**ersistent **H**allucination, **N**egative symptoms, **I**ncoherence, **C**atatonic features. There are further criteria for each sub-type of schizophrenia.

OSCE 13 – History

Actor instructions
You appear unhappy, particularly about your current social situation, but logical and willing to talk. You reveal more unprompted information when asked open questions and not interrupted.

You talk about your depressive symptoms more readily than your psychotic ones, which you hint at but don't explicitly mention unless specifically asked.

When asked about	You mention
Your name	My name is Kurdt Fraser, Kurdt with a "d".
Presenting complaint	I am currently feeling down. Things have not been going well for me. I used to work as a maths teacher, but they got rid of me because of my illness. That was 2 months ago, it started another 2 months before that. I couldn't pay my rent, so I moved back with my parents. I'm not sleeping properly and I want to move out, but there are so many things for me to sort out first, like getting a job. The only money I've got coming in at the moment is the occasional bit of A-level tuition.
Your mood	I just feel very down, like I can't do anything, like anything I do makes things worse. I don't have the energy, especially in the mornings. When it gets like this, there's nothing that seems interesting.
Self-harm	Four years ago, I slit my wrists and had to go to the hospital, but it wasn't serious. I'm not thinking about killing myself these days.
Hearing voices	Sometimes I hear voices, calling me idiot and fool. They've told me to kill myself before and I've heard news reports about me causing a plane crash in Peru, saying the police were looking for me. Sometimes they tell me that medication is

government mind control but I know it's dangerous to stop. I'm not hearing voices now though.

Seeing special signs   I've never had anything like that.

Control of your thoughts   There have been times when I've felt that people around me could hear my thoughts. Especially my family. But this hasn't been happening in the last few months.

Control of your actions   I've always felt in control, apart from when I hear the voices telling me stuff, but even then I know I can choose what to do.

Past psychiatric history   I've been sectioned twice before. I get paranoid sometimes, about my family trying to wipe me out. I first started getting paranoid when I was 21, but I think my depression came on first. The paranoid feelings and the depression, they both come and go. It's been that way since the last 7 years, both problems are about the same intensity.

Past medical history   My appendix burst when I was 13. Other than that, I have had no serious illnesses.

Drug use   I have never tried drugs. I don't drink.

Medication   I have been on many medications for my psychiatric problems. Currently I am on citalopram and olanzapine, but have been tried on paroxetine and risperidone, amongst others.

Family history   My mother and father are very healthy, touch wood. They have not had psychiatric problems. I have 2 brothers, and they are also healthy.

Marking Scheme	
2 marks: Good - 1 mark: Adequate - 0 mark: Poor/Not done	**Mark 0 – 2**
1. Polite introduction. Verifies identity.	☐
2. Finds duration of symptoms.	☐
3. Elicits past psychiatric history.	☐
4. Asks about auditory hallucinations.	☐
5. Asks about delusions of thought control.	☐
6. Asks about delusions of passivity.	☐
7. Asks about delusions of perception.	☐
8. Elicits depressive features: ▪ low mood	☐
9. ▪ anergia	☐
10. ▪ anhedonia	☐
11. ▪ sleep disturbance	☐
12. Asks about deliberate self harm.	☐
13. Elicits past medical history.	☐
14. Asks about drug abuse.	☐
15, Elicits drug history.	☐
16. Elicits family history.	☐
17. Thanks the patient. Overall impression.	☐
Examiner's additional questions (near the end)	
Q: What is the diagnosis?	
18. **A:** Schizoaffective disorder/ depression with psychosis. (1 mark for schizophrenia)	☐
TOTAL SCORE	**/ 36**

Further information

Schizoaffective disorder is diagnosed when illness fitting the criteria of schizophrenia occurs with depression or mania, providing that both aspects are of the same intensity. Psychotic and affective symptoms may occur simultaneously or alternate. Schizoaffective disorder lifetime prevalence is ~1 per 200 people, typically starting in the early twenties or late teens. Schizoaffective treatment consists of talking therapies and antipsychotic medication combined with antidepressants or mood stabilizers as required. The rate of relapse rate can be as high as 50-60% in adverse circumstances, but with family support (including reducing the level of expressed emotion), this may fall to ~10%. 30-40% are said to attempt suicide, with ~10% succeeding.

OSCE 14 – History

Actor instruction
You are playing the role of a GP, calling a junior doctor about one of your patients.

You volunteer this first piece of information:

"Hello this is Dr Sanderson, I am phoning about my patient Kerry Johnson. Kerry is 22 and was diagnosed as schizophrenic 2 years ago. Her mother just called me, saying Kerry is furious and has not been taking her medication. She becomes very upset when her mother approaches and has locked herself in the garden shed. She accuses her mother of poisoning her."

For any other information, wait for the doctor to ask you specifically.

When asked about	You mention
Risk assessment	She has no history of self harm or violence to others, but her mother is worried because Kerry has a knife and is threatening to cut herself if she approaches.
Previous compulsory admissions	She has had one compulsory admission, 18 months ago, which lasted 28 days.
Your opinion	I think this is serious and Kerry needs to be admitted.
The family's view	Kerry's mother is very worried and wants her to be admitted to a psychiatric unit.
If you have any questions	<ul><li>What section is most appropriate in this case?</li><li>Who is the applicant for this section?</li><li>Which healthcare worker can sign this section?</li><li>How long does this section last?</li><li>What is the appeal procedure for this section?</li></ul>

Marking Scheme	
2 marks: Good - 1 mark: Adequate - 0 mark: Poor/Not done	**Mark 0 – 2**

1. Polite introduction. ☐
2. Listens to scenario. ☐
3. Asks about previous admissions. ☐
4. Asks about risk assessment, including deliberate self harm and harm to others. ☐
5. Asks what GP thinks is appropriate. ☐
6. Asks about view of patient's family. ☐
7. Section 4, emergency admission, is most appropriate. ☐
8. Applicant is nearest relative or an approved social worker. ☐
9. A doctor of any rank can sign section 4. ☐
10. A section 4 admission lasts 72 hours. ☐
11. There isn't an appeals process for a section 4. ☐
12. Overall impression. ☐

TOTAL SCORE   **/ 24**

Further information

People in need of psychiatric treatment, particularly when a danger to themselves or others, and refusing or incapable of giving consent, can be compulsorily admitted under the 1983 Mental Health Act (in England and Wales). Applications are made to the managers of a hospital. The responsible medical officer (RMO) may terminate any compulsory admission before the prescribed period of detention. While detained under the mental health act, patients are allow to marry, but can't vote; other activities may be allowed, dependent on their capacity. Patients may have one review tribunal during their admission, and have an automatic hearing after 6 months stay. A patient has unlimited appeals to a manager's meeting, the panel consisting of non-executive hospital directors. The Mental Health Act commission inspects the administration and operation of the act.

Examples of compulsory civil admissions are given below. When 2 doctors are required to sign, they must be independent, working at different sites. Drug treatment beyond 3 months requires consent or a second opinion. In the UK, there are plans to broaden the criteria for admission and reduce the right to appeal.

Part II of the Mental Health Act 1983 - Compulsory Admission Procedures

Section	Signatories	Applicant	Duration	Manner of termination
Section 2: Admission for assessment	2 doctors, one of whom is approved	Nearest relative or an approved social worker	28 days	1. Patient discharged or remains informally. 2. Application for section 3. Appeal possible by patient application for Mental health review tribunal or managers meeting.
Section 3: Admission for treatment	2 doctors, one of whom is approved	Nearest relative or an approved social worker	6 months, renewable for a further 6 months and then at yearly intervals	1. Patient discharged or remains informally. 2. Discharged by the nearest relative unless barred by RMO. Appeal possible by application for mental health tribunal by patient or nearest relative or automatic manager's meeting after 6 months.
Section 4: Emergency admission	Any doctor	Nearest relative or an approved social worker	72 hours	1. Patient discharged or remains informally. 2. Regraded to section 2 or application for section 3.
Section 5(2): Emergency detention of informal patient	The doctor in charge or his nominated deputy	None	72 hours	1. Patient discharged or remains informally. 2. regarded to section 2 or application for section 3 initiated.
Section 5(4): Nurses holding power for informal patients	A first-level trained nurse	None	6 hours	1. Patient discharged or remains informally. 2. Section 5(2) applied by doctor.

OSCE 15 – Explaining lithium treatment

Actor instructions

You are talkative and mention your history with little prompting. Provided the information is explained clearly, you have no problem describing its main risks and benefits when asked.

Examiner has a lithium leaflet which they hand over when it is mentioned.

When asked about	You mention
Your name	I'm Gina Headley.
Your condition	4 weeks ago they diagnosed me with bipolar. I didn't want no medication at first because I've heard it's dangerous, plus I was worried I might lose my edge. I work in admin and as a comedy writer and performer. And also I'm studying my second year of an Open University degree in Maths. People even said to me stuff like "Maybe you should get some help" but I thought they were just saying I was funny! I didn't mind! I thought it was a compliment. Now, though, the bipolar is making it harder to keep all these plates spinning, you know?
Self-harm	I have never self-harmed. I think self-harming is wrong, because no matter how low you get, you shouldn't need to end it all, that's too much.
Past medical history	As far back as I can remember, I've always been a healthy person. Apart from having this bipolar, what do you call it, psychiatrically challenged? But seriously, my health has been decent.
Drug history	I was given paroxetine when I was on a depression. I think this made my bipolar worse. I started on olanzapine 3 days ago for the bipolar, other than that I'm not on anything, not even the pill.
Substance abuse	I haven't taken any drugs for more than 4 years. My friends used to do coke and I used to take it

too, especially when I was depressed. That was stupid, yeah, cos it didn't help much. I've given up alcohol as well and I don't smoke.

If you have any questions
- Would lithium be safe in pregnancy?
- Also, how long does it take to work?
- How safe is lithium?

Consent
On balance, I would be willing to go ahead.

Marking Scheme	
2 marks: Good - 1 mark: Adequate - 0 mark: Poor/Not done	**Mark 0 – 2**

1. Polite introduction. Checks patient's identity. ☐
2. Elicits history of bipolar disorder. ☐
3. Asks about self-harm. ☐
4. Asks about past medical history. ☐
5. Takes drug history. ☐
6. Asks about substance abuse. ☐
7. Basic explanation of drug mechanism e.g. stabilizes excitable neurons that cause mania. ☐
8. Explains treatment likely to be long-term, with danger of relapse on sudden cessation. ☐
9. Underlines risk of overdose due to narrow therapeutic margin. ☐
10. Explains common side-effects- mild tremor, metallic taste, increased urination, tiredness, vomiting. ☐
11. Explains serious side-effects that could require dose reduction/ termination e.g. severe GI disturbances, hypothyroidism, and dehydration. ☐
12. Explains hypothyroidism symptoms to look out for e.g. goitre, oedema, weight gain, cold intolerance, anergia, reduced concentration. ☐
13. Explains diabetes insipidus symptoms to look out for polyuria, polydipsia, dehydration. ☐
14. Explains which blood tests and physical checks required before initiation. ☐
15. Explains which blood tests are required with maintenance. Asks for questions. ☐

16. Explains that lithium is best avoided when trying for a baby, during pregnancy & breast-feeding due to the risk of cardiac defects. Therefore she needs reliable contraception and should tell her doctors when she is planning a pregnancy. □

17. Explains most people respond in 2 weeks, but may need up to 6 weeks. □

18. Explains lithium is relatively safe and effective though monitoring plus precautions are required, with reviews in future about continuing use. □

19. Explains lithium red card system. □

20. Mentions a leaflet is available (at which point examiner hands it to her). □

21. Checks understanding and asks for consent in a non-coercive fashion. □

22. Overall impression. □

TOTAL SCORE **/ 44**

Further information

This station involves taking a brief history from a talkative patient, leaving enough time for explanation. The brief history is relevant due to the risk of overdose; specialist input is required before starting long-term lithium prophylaxis. Lithium is thought to work by stabilizing serotonin receptors in the prefrontal cortex. It is most effective during the manic phase, doesn't risk causing depression and has relatively minor effects on cognition. Once the initial effects are experienced, people may feel "cured" and thus non-compliance is a major problem, especially since the drug may not be effective after a relapse. If a manic patient is taking antidepressants, these should be stopped, at a rate that avoids withdrawal symptoms. Acute mania is often initially treated with atypical antipsychotics alongside lithium because the latter takes days to work. Patients must be informed of its side-effects and the risks of stopping early; the need for contraception should be explicitly discussed with all women of childbearing age. Maintenance therapy is generally only started when the patient has a second manic episode; with a first-line prophylactic agent like lithium, olanzapine or valproate (NICE 2006). Suicide risk in bipolar affective disorder may be as high as 10-15%.

OSCE 16 – History

Actor instructions

You look at the floor and appear tired; your responses are based on the replies below. You speak slowly and volunteer little information, leaving silent gaps after your terse answers.

When asked about	You mention
Your name	Hello my name is Waheeda Qureishi.
Your mood	I've been feeling down for the last few weeks, tired all the time. Pretty down about myself, the way things have been going.
Mood variation during the day	I feel worse during the morning. I don't feel like getting up.
Early morning waking	I wake up early and can't get back to sleep.
Loss of pleasure	I've lost interest in badminton. I can't concentrate at work. Even trying to read a magazine, my mind wanders and I can't focus. I don't feel like reading books or listening to music. I don't feel like seeing my friends or family, I can't face it at the moment.
Suicide	I've not even thought about it.
Weight loss	I've been losing weight, I miss meals.
Previous psychiatric history	I've never been depressed before.
Hallucinations	I've never heard voices before.
Previous elevated mood	I've never had phases of feeling unusually happy.
Preceding events	At work, there's been some politics, the usual rubbish. It's been stressful for the last 4 months. I don't really want to go into it, sorry.

Motor problems   I've not had any shakes or particular slowness.

**Home circum-
stances**   I live with my husband and daughter. I haven't been getting on with my husband or my parents so well. He says I should work more hours. He says I'm lazy. My daughter is at primary school, I try and keep all this away from her but I think she realises.

Guilt   I don't feel good about it do I? But it's an illness, that's what I think, so it's not something I control.

General Health   I'm alright medically, I've never even had a serious illness.

Medication   I have never taken medication.

Drug use   I've never taken drugs, I don't drink.

Marking Scheme	
2 marks: Good - 1 mark: Adequate - 0 mark: Poor/Not done	**Mark 0 – 2**

1. Polite introduction. Verifies identity.
2. Finds out about mood and its variation through the day.
3. Finds out about low self-esteem.
4. Finds out about biological symptoms ▪ Weight loss
5. ▪ Early morning waking
6. ▪ Loss of energy
7. ▪ Loss of concentration
8. Asks about suicidal thoughts.
9. Asks about motor symptoms.
10. Asks about guilt.
11. Asks about medical history.
12. Excludes previous history of psychosis.
13. Excludes previous history of mania.
14. Asks about drug history.
15. Asks about drug abuse.
16. Thanks the patient. Overall impression.

Examiner's additional questions (near the end)	
Q: What is the diagnosis?	
17. **A:** Depression.	☐
Q: What is the severity?	
18. **A:** Moderate. (See 6 features below)	☐

TOTAL SCORE	**/ 36**

Further information

Depression is thought to occur when unhappiness is sustained for longer than expected, disproportionate to adverse circumstances and with significant impairment of daily functioning. A WHO study found that ~10% of patients consulting their GP could be classed as having an ICD-10 depressive episode. Depression may cause somatic features, such as appetite disturbance, sleep disorder and impairment of concentration. Genetic influences are most marked in severe depression. Brown and Harris (1979) found that adverse life events were more likely to cause depression in women with 4 vulnerability factors: absence of a close confiding friend or partner, loss of their mother before they reached 11 years of age, lack of employment outside the home, 3 or more children aged less than 15 living with them. Working-class women were more likely to experience adverse events and to have more vulnerability factors, which Brown and Harris surmised impaired self-esteem and coping skills, explaining their greater depression prevalence compared to professional women. Depression is approximately twice as common amongst women, with other contributory factors including being post-partum.

ICD-10 depression criteria (duration at least 2 weeks, not due to organic, drug, psychotic or bereavement disorder)
a) Low mood most of the day.
b) Anhedonia (loss of pleasure).
c) Anergia (loss of energy with increased fatigability).
d) Significant weight loss/gain or appetite change.
e) Sleep disturbance (typically early morning waking)
f) Psychomotor agitation or retardation
g) Low self-esteem and self-confidence
h) Excessive and disproportionate feelings of guilt and unworthiness.
i) Diminished concentration
j) Recurrent suicidal ideation, recurrent thoughts of death or actual suicide attempt or plan.

Severity criteria for depression

Dysthymia: less than 4 of the above or less than 2 of a) to c); not as severe as depression but may last longer.

Mild depression: at least 2 of a) to c) and 2-3 of d) to i).

Moderate depression: at least 2 of a) to c) and enough of d) to i) for a total of 6-7 features.

Severe depression: a), b) and c) plus at least 5 of d) to i). Usual activities have ceased and basic self-care is compromised, with a high risk of suicide (~15%). Depression featuring psychosis (mood-congruent) or stupor is always considered severe.

These features can be remembered by the mnemonic **DEAD SWAMP** (de Beer 2001)- **D**epressed mood, **E**nergy loss, **A**nhedonia, thoughts of **D**eath, **S**leep disturbances, **W**orthlessness or excessive guilt, **A**ppetite or weight change, **M**entation impaired, **P**sychomotor agitation or retardation.

	Depressive features
Appearance	Possible weight loss, blunted affect, self-neglect.
Behaviour	Psychomotor agitation/ retardation, poor eye contact.
Cognition	Reduced attention and concentration, which can cause depressive pseudodementia.
Speech	May have poverty of speech.
Thought	Beck's cognitive triad- negative view of self (guilt), negative view of the world (negative interpretation of day-to-day events), hopeless view of the future.
Insight	Normally intact, unless mood-congruent delusions e.g. delusions of ill-health, guilt, worthlessness, persecution, nihilism (Cotard's syndrome)
Mood	Unhappy or numb.
Perceptions	Normal, unless mood-congruent hallucination (mainly auditory)

OSCE 17 – Fitness to plead

Actor instructions

You have a mild learning disability, but live an independent life. If the student uses jargon or over-long questions you respond "pardon me?" You reveal more when asked open questions.

When asked about	You mention
Your name	I am Ken Larkins.
What happened	I was in the pub last night. I was with my friends, and this guy came up to me shouting. He said I spilt his beer. I didn't spill his beer. He got louder and louder. He called me names and all his mates laughed. That's when I lamped him one dead on the jaw. He was bigger than me and all, went down, smack, straight away. I didn't kick him, I made sure my mates didn't kick him because that's not what I'm like. His mates were laughing before but where did they go? They scattered. He got up, everyone staring so obviously he had to hit me back. He tried coming at me with a bottle, but I kicked him in the head this time and he went down again. My mate said jump on his head, but I didn't want to. The second time he come at me, I stepped inside his punch, then headbutted him. I think that's how he broke his nose. But after that, I left, I didn't want anything more to do with it.
How much you drank	I don't drink alcohol, I just go to the pub for the company.
Previous court experience	I've never been in trouble with the law before.
Understanding of court procedure	I've seen it on TV. The judge sits up high, everyone listens to him, call him "your honour" and "sir". The defence lawyer supports you, the prosecution tries to prove you're lying.

If you know what you have been charged with	Assault, attacking someone for no reason.
If you did anything wrong	Not really. I wish I hadn't hurt him, but he started it, ask anyone that was there. He shouldn't bother people.
if you understand guilty and non-guilty pleas	I'll plead not guilty, because he provoked me and then tried to kill me.
If you think you could instruct a lawyer	I've spoken to him already, he agrees with me.

Marking Scheme	
2 marks: Good - 1 mark: Adequate - 0 mark: Poor/Not done	**Mark 0 – 2**
1. Polite introduction. Verifies identity.	☐
2. Gets the patient's version of events.	☐
3. Asks how much he had drunk.	☐
4. Asks about previous court experience.	☐
5. Asks about understanding of court procedure.	☐
6. Asks if he knows what he's been charged with.	☐
7. Asks if they know why they have been charged.	☐
8. Asks if they know the difference between pleading guilty and not guilty.	☐
9 Asks if they know how to instruct counsel.	☐
10. Overall impression	☐
Examiner's additional questions (near the end)	
Q: Is the patient fit to plead?	
11. A: Yes	☐
TOTAL SCORE	**/ 22**

Further information

To be fit to enter a plea, a person must be able to:

- Understand the nature of the charge.
- Understand the difference between guilty and not guilty pleas.
- Instruct lawyers.
- Follow court proceedings sufficiently to challenge jurors.

Fitness to plead is based on the defendant's state of mind at the time of the trial. It is decided by a jury based on psychiatric evidence. If a defendant is deemed unfit, in their absence a second jury is called for a **"trial of facts"**. This can result in discharge or hospital detention.

Diminished responsibility refers solely to murder charges; when a guilty verdict is reached, it is deemed manslaughter not murder. A **plea of insanity** requires that during the offence, the defendant was so mentally ill that they were unaware what they were doing, or if they were aware, that they couldn't tell it was wrong.

Pleas of insanity are dealt with by the Criminal Procedure (Insanity and Unfitness to Plead) Act 1991. **Infanticide** is the killing by violence or neglect by a woman of her child aged less than 12 months, while in a disturbed state of mind (e.g. puerperal psychosis); the court can pass any sentence.

Automatism refers to actions without conscious intent and is described as **"insane"** or **"sane"**. Insane automatism is judged likely to recur and has adjudged "internal" causes such as somnambulism, with indeterminate detention permitted. Sane automatism refers to one-off events, said to have "external" causes such as hypoglycaemia or concussion, and if proven, leads to acquittal.

OSCE 18 – Discussing antidepressant therapy

Actor instructions
You are tired and defensive; your responses are based on the replies below. You reveal more unprompted information when asked open questions and not interrupted.

Examiner has a leaflet which they produce when it is mentioned by the student.

When asked about	You mention
Your name	I'm Richard Harmon.
What you feel about antidepressants	The main reason I don't want to take your antidepressants is that I don't think I'm depressed. I've made mistakes and now it's up to me to sort them out my way. It was on the news, seroxat, it can make you climb the walls, cut yourself and all sorts. Frankly I resent the way they're being pushed on me.
Your symptoms	I've been feeling down for the last 2 months, not enjoying anything. I'm really tired because I haven't been sleeping. I've been losing weight, losing concentration and I've been off work for 1 week.
Suicide	I've been thinking about it though, just coming into my mind. I wouldn't overdose on medication though.
If you have any questions	▪ What are the side-effects? ▪ How likely are they to work? ▪ What happens if they don't work? ▪ How long do I have to take them? ▪ Can I have any other kind of treatment?

Marking Scheme	
2 marks: Good - 1 mark: Adequate - 0 mark: Poor/Not done	**Mark 0 – 2**
1. Polite introduction. Verifies identity.	☐
2. Explains what they are about to do and asks permission.	☐
3. Takes reconciliatory tone- e.g. acknowledging his anger, saying no one will try to force him into taking drugs.	☐
4. Asks about depressive symptoms.	☐
5. Assesses suicidality.	☐
6. Explains depression is an acknowledged illness.	☐
7. Explains drug mechanisms e.g. depression associated with reduced levels of brain chemicals which antidepressants can increase, with effects versus moderate to severe depression.	☐
8. Asks the patient he has any questions.	☐
9. Explains that side-effects would be monitored regularly, doses can be varied or regimen changed according to tolerance. E.g. tricyclics may cause drowsiness and rarely arrhythmias, while selective serotonin reuptake inhibitors can sometimes cause diarrhoea and short-lived increases in anxiety but are safer in overdose.	☐
10. Explains that there is no guarantee but most patients with moderate to severe depression are substantially improved within 3 months of starting treatment.	☐
11. Explains that treatment should be maintained for ~ 4 weeks before response is assessed: effects take time. If treatment doesn't work, doses are tapered off gradually, and new options explored- drugs +/- psychological approaches.	☐
12. Explains that if treatment alleviates depression it should be be for a minimum of 6 months, with gradual tapering over 4-6 weeks- suddenly stopping causes rebound depression.	☐
13. Explains non-medical treatments e.g. cognitive behavioural or interpersonal therapy.	☐
14. Offers a leaflet or mentions a relevant depression group.	☐
15. Overall impression.	☐
TOTAL SCORE	**/ 30**

Further information
There have been concerns raised about the number of people in the UK taking antidepressants, particularly when their problems are largely social in origin. However, antidepressants are considered safe and effective treatment when used appropriately, though they are not recommended for mild depression. In 2003, the Committee on Safety of Medicines (CSM) advised that the SSRI's citalopram, escitalopram, paroxetine, and sertraline, alongside other antidepressants mirtazepine and venlafaxine should not be given to those under 18, due to an increased risk of self-harm and suicidal behaviour.

While studies have proved the efficacy of cognitive behavioural therapy, it isn't always available and waiting lists tend to be long. Other non-drug approaches include interpersonal therapy, problem-solving therapy, social interventions and self-help groups. Cognitive behavioural therapy tends to be given in short-term programmes, focused on specific problems, identifying thought patterns that contribute to their low mood.

OSCE 19 – History

Actor instructions
You are withdrawn and quiet; your answers are based on the responses below. You reveal more unprompted information when asked open questions and not interrupted.

When asked about	You mention
Your name	I'm Belinda Robertson.
What happened	Tonight was a really bad night for me. I'd been planning this for weeks. My flatmate was out and I locked myself in my room. I took maybe 40 paracetamols. I didn't realise my mum would call. I was half-conscious and I could hear ringing, but I didn't pick up. She realized something was wrong, came round knocking on the door, got no answer, somehow got the neighbour to kick it down, then kick down my bedroom door. I wasn't happy when I woke up.
Why you took the paracetamol	I've been down for a while. I've got a little boy that's 6 years old and they took him away and I've not got access. My babyfather's dead, he died 3 years ago today in a car crash. I'd been thinking a lot about it. I didn't see anything for me in the future.
If you wrote a note	I wrote a note to my mum, to my daughter and one to my little sister.
If you would do it again	I still feel the same way about things, I'd probably try it again.
If you attempted suicide before	I've been admitted for heroin overdoses but none of them were deliberate.
Drug history	I was addicted to heroin for 6 years, been clean for more than 2. I don't smoke or drink alcohol anymore either. I did well at school, you know. My boyfriend was an addict, he got me into it,

but not like he put a gun to my head. First it was smoking smack, then injecting. I ripped off my family and all my friends, did other things for money.

If you hear any voices   I don't hear any voices like that.
from people that
aren't there

If you feel your   No.
thoughts are controlled
by outside forces

Family history   My mother's the only one that's stuck by me. I haven't seen my dad in years. No one else in the family is like me. I don't know anyone who's killed themselves.

Marking Scheme	
2 marks: Good - 1 mark: Adequate - 0 mark: Poor/Not done	**Mark 0 – 2**
1. Polite introduction, verifies identity, establishes rapport.	☐
2. Finds reasons for attempted suicide.	☐
3. Assesses suicidal intent: ▪ when no one is at home	☐
4. ▪ planned in advance	☐
5. ▪ wrote notes	☐
6. ▪ current feelings	☐
7. Asks about previous suicide attempts.	☐
8. Asks about family history.	☐
9 Asks about drug history.	☐
10. Asks about auditory hallucinations.	☐
11. Asks about delusions of thought control.	☐
12. Overall empathetic approach.	☐
Examiner's additional questions (near the end)	
Q: Should the patient be admitted? Why? 13. **A:** Patient needs to be admitted for treatment of overdose and to prevent her attempting suicide again.	☐
TOTAL SCORE	**/ 26**

Further information
Risk factors for suicide include previous attempts, mental illness (~15% lifetime risk with severe depression, ~10% with schizophrenia), family history, alcohol and drug abuse, having a painful or terminal illness, having access to poisons or weapons (e.g. farmers) and social stressors (e.g. imprisonment).

Suicide in the UK accounts for ~1% of all deaths. Intent is assessed by asking about a history of self-harm, why they did it, current thoughts about previous suicide attempts/self-harm, current mood level, and any suicide plans made such as method and notes written. Attempting suicide while intoxicated and/or surrounded by people who could intervene indicates a lesser intent than doing so alone after months of sober deliberation.

Methods such as drug overdose and severing veins are potentially fatal but less certain to kill than jumping under a train or severing an artery. The greater the planning and intention, the more precautions are required, with supervised admission for those at highest risk.

OSCE 20 – History

Actor instructions
You are quiet and lethargic. You talk reluctantly about painful episodes and make little eye contact. You speak less if many questions are asked and are more likely to answer following periods of silence.

When asked about	You mention
Your name	Hello I'm Kelly Weaver.
Your mood	About two months ago, my mother then my husband died, within one week of each other.
What happened	My mother was 71. She caught pneumonia, and she went quite fast. She'd been in poor health for a while. My husband was only a year older than me. He was driving at night and smoke started coming out of the bonnet, so he pulled over. He was waiting on the hard shoulder when his car got hit by a lorry. We've got 2 kids, a boy and a girl. I took a week off work, then I went back, but it was too much. I've been losing interest in everything.
Sleep	It's hard to get a decent sleep. I tend to wake up early as well and then I can't fall asleep again. Most days I cry first thing I wake up. I see him sometimes when I'm about to drop off. My mum too sometimes. I used to see them when I was awake too, does that mean I'm losing it?
Effect on your life	My family's been really great, they help me look after them, bring meals. But I don't think they expected me to react like this. I haven't been to work for a month. My son's getting bullied at school. I feel like I'm letting them down. They're warming up food for me, going out to buy me fags, it's not fair. I should have taken the car to the garage then it wouldn't have happened. I used to talk to my mum all the time.

Weight loss	I've lost more than 2 stone in 2 months.
What you were like before	This time 6 months ago, I was a completely different woman. I've never been depressed before. I could never foresee this, you know?
Your view of the future	It's not good. I can't see much light.
Suicide	I've definitely thought about killing myself. But I couldn't do that to my kids.
Medication	My GP said I could go on antidepressants, but I didn't want to.
Alcohol use	I've been drinking. Maybe 4 or 5 shots of whisky per day. It helps to sleep. I've been smoking more, maybe 20 per day.
Drug use	Last week, a friend of mine gave me some cannabis. Then she said to try ketamine, but I've stopped now because it wasn't helping.

Marking Scheme

2 marks: Good - 1 mark: Adequate - 0 mark: Poor/Not done	Mark 0 – 2
1. Polite introduction. Verifies identity.	☐
2. Explains what they are about to do and asks permission.	☐
3. Finds duration of symptoms and precipitating events.	☐
4. Asks about appetite.	☐
5. Asks about sleeping.	☐
6. Finds out about anhedonia and lethargy.	☐
7. Asks about her view of the future.	☐
8. Asks about premorbid personality.	☐
9. Excludes history of previous mental illness.	☐
10 Asks about medication.	☐
11. Asks about alcohol use.	☐

12. Asks about drug use. ☐
13. Asks about suicide. ☐
14. Assures her that it is normal to glimpse departed loved ones ☐
    after bereavement.
15. Overall empathetic approach. ☐

Examiner's additional questions (near the end)

Q: What is the diagnosis?
16. **A:** Reactive depression following bereavement. ☐

Q: What treatment options are there?
17. **A:** Bereavement counselling and/or antidepressants. ☐

TOTAL SCORE / 34

Further information
The process of grief can be divided into 3 stages: denial, sadness and acceptance, which are not necessarily sequential. Denial may last from hours to days, often with a numb lack of emotional response. The second stage is characterised by poor sleep, social withdrawal, reduced appetite, clinging to memories, guilt and blame. Imagery, illusions, hallucinations and felt presences of the departed are commonly felt during bereavement, and it can help if they are warned about beforehand. During resolution, social contact increases and happy memories are retained, though the sadness may return at anniversaries. It may be useful to explain this potentially cyclical process.

Pathological grief tends to have a later onset, last longer than 6 months, and be more intense. It is more likely when the death was sudden and the person has difficulty showing their emotions, perhaps because of caring for their children. When pathological grief is suspected, antidepressant therapy should be discussed; counselling, support groups and assistance dealing with practical problems such as funeral arrangements may also help. To achieve a sense of finality, it may be of benefit for them to see the body and put away the dead person's possessions. As they progress into acceptance, they may respond to encouragement to renew social contact, while trying to hold onto happy memories.

11 Abbreviations

ABG	Arterial blood gas
ACTH	Adrenocorticotrophin
BCG	Bacille Calmette-Guérin (live attenuated tuberculosis vaccine)
CBT	Cognitive behavioural therapy
CK	Creatine kinase
CMV	Cytomegalovirus
CNS	Central nervous system (brain and spinal cord)
CRH	Corticotrophin releasing hormone
CSF	Cerebrospinal fluid
CT	Computer tomography
CVA	Cerebrovascular accident
DVLA	Driver and Vehicle Licensing Agency
ECG	Electrocardiogram
EEG	Electroencephalogram
Elispot	Enzyme-linked immunosorbent spot, finds T cells primed to Mycobacterium Tuberculosis
EMG	Electromyogram
ESR	Erythrocyte Sedimentation Rate, in mm/hour. This is abnormal if greater than (age+10)/2 in women, or greater than age/2 in men.
	FBC Full blood count
FSH	Follicle stimulating hormone
GBS	Guillain-Barré syndrome
GH	Growth Hormone
H. Influenzae	Haemophilus Influenzae
5-HT	5-hydroxytryptamine
IV	Intravenous
LH	Luteinising hormone
LFT	Liver function test
LMN	Lower motor neurone
Meningococcus	Neisseria meningitidis
MMR	Measles mumps and rubella vaccination

MPTP	1-methyl 4-phenyl 1,2,3,6-tetrahydropyridine (a designer drug which causes rapid basal ganglia damage and Parkinsonian symptoms)
MRI	Magnetic resonance imaging
MS	Multiple sclerosis
M.Tuberculosis	Mycobacterium tuberculosis
PAG	Periaqueductal grey
PCR	Polymerase chain reaction
PET	Positron emission tomography (displays the metabolic activity of brain regions)
SSRIs	Selective serotonin reuptake inhibitors
TFT	Thyroid function test
TSH	Thyroid stimulating hormone
U&E	Urea and electrolytes
UMN	Upper motor neurone
WHO	World Health Organisation

12 Mnemonics

TOPIC	MNEMONIC/ Memory tool	MEANING
Alcohol abuse screening questionnaire	CAGE	Ever tried to Cut down? Annoyed when people tell you to cut down? Ever feel Guilty about drinking? Ever have an Eye-cap (drink on waking)? 2 or more positive answers suggest further enquiry regarding alcohol intake and possible dependency.
Ankylosing spondylitis (Features)	8 As	Anterior uveitis, Apical lung fibrosis, Aortic regurgitation, AV node block, Amyloidosis, Atlanto-axial subluxation, Achilles tendonitis, Axial arthritis.
Anorexia nervosa (ICD-10 criteria)	WEIgheD	Weight reduced (BMI <17.5kg/m² or less than 85% expected weight), Endocrine disturbance, overvalued Idea (dread of being obesity, belief they are overweight), Deliberate weight loss [all 4 required].
Argyll Robertson pupil	ARP forwards PRA backwards	Accommodation Response Present, Pupillary Response Absent
Aspects of disease	Doctors ARe Always Emphasising History and Examination In Management of Clinical Problems	Definition, Differential diagnoses, At Risk (risk factors), Aetiology, Epidemiology, History and Examination (clinical features), Investigation results, Management, Complications, Prognosis.
Carpal Tunnel Syndrome (Tests)	Tinel-Tap, Phalen-Flexion	Tinel's and Phalen's are tests for carpal tunnel syndrome. Tinel's involves tapping over the palmar surface of the wrist, Phalen's involves holding the wrist in flexion.
Cerebellar disease (Signs)	DANISH	Dysdiadochokinesis, Ataxia, Nystagmus, Intention tremor, Slurred or Staccato speech (can't enunciate "British Constitution"), Hypotonia.

TOPIC	MNEMONIC/ Memory tool	MEANING
12 cranial nerves	On Old Olympus Towering Tops, A Finn And German Viewed Some Hops (Gupta '98)	Olfactory, Optic, Oculomotor, Trochlear, Trigeminal, Abducens, Facial, Vestibulocochlear, Glosso-pharyngeal, Vagus, Accessory, Hy-poglossal
Depression (ICD-10 criteria)	DEAD SWAMP (de Beer 2001)	Depressed mood, Energy loss, Anhe-donia, thoughts of Death, Sleep dis-turbances, Worthlessness or exces-sive guilt, Appetite or weight change, Mentation impaired, Psychomotor agitation or retardation [Minimum 4, duration at least 2 weeks].
Disease mechanisms (Checklist)	INVITE MItCH Down	Infection, Neoplasm, Vascular, auto-Immune, Trauma, Endocrine, Meta-bolic, Idiopathic, Congenital, Haema-tological, Drug-related, Degenerative
Gerstmann syndrome (Clinical features)	AALF	Alexia, Acalulia, Left-right disorienta-tion, Finger agnosia (dominant parie-tal lesion)
Hearing loss (Clinical features of conductive and sensorineural)	Weber -- Wally Rinné -- Ringing in ears	In Weber's test, tuning fork is placed on forehead, making person resem-ble a Wally. In Rinne's test, tuning fork is placed outside external mea-tus, ringing in ears.
Hormones released from anterior pituitary	GP SAT	Growth hormone, Prolactin, Sex hor-mones (LH and FSH), ACTH, TSH
Intrinsic muscles of hand (Nerve supply to)	LOAF	Intrinsic muscles of the hand sup-plied by median nerve- 2 lateral Lumbricals, Opponens pollicis, Ab-ductor pollicis brevis and Flexor pol-licis brevis (all the rest supplied by ulnar nerve).
Mania without psy-chosis (ICD-10 crite-ria)	GRAnDIoSITy	Grandiosity or inflated self-esteem, Reckless behavior, increased Activi-ty, Distractibility and Disinbition, In-somnia, marked Sexual energy, flight of Ideas, increased Talkativeness [3+ required, 4+ if mood is irritable not elated, lasting at least 1 week].
Neurological exam (Components)	ATP RSC (Eves 2004)	Appearance, Tone, Power, Reflexes, Sensation, Coordination (Eves 2004)
Optic nerve examina-tion	AFRO	Acuity, Fields, Reflexes, Ophthalmo-scopy

TOPIC	MNEMONIC/ Memory tool	MEANING
Pain history	SOCRATES	Site, Onset, Character, Radiation, Alleviating factors, Timing, Exacerbating factors, Severity
Parkinson's disease (Signs)	TRAPS	Tremor, Rigidity, Akinesia, Postural instability, Shuffling gait
Peripheral neuropathy (Causes)	A to H	Alcohol, B12 deficiency, Cancer + Connective tissue diseases, Diabetes + Drugs (e.g. phenytoin), Everything else (e.g. vasculitis), Friedrich's ataxia, Guillain-Barré syndrome, Hereditary motor-sensory neuropathy (Charcot-Marie-Toooth syndrome)
Psychiatric mental state examination (Components)	ABC RST IMP	ABC (Appearance, Behaviour, Cognition), RST (Rapport, Speech, Thought pattern), IMP (Insight, Mood, Perception
Ring-enhancing CT brain lesions (Causes)	MAGIC DR	Metastases, Abscesses, Glioma and other primary brain tumours, Infarction, Contusion, De-myelination, Resolving haematoma
Schizophrenia (ICD-10 criteria)	sCHIZ	Group 1- Control/passivity, auditory Hallucinations in 1st or 3rd person, thought Insertion/ withdrawal/ broadcast, biZarre delusions
	OPHreNIC	Group 2- Other Persistent Hallucination, Negative symptoms, Incoherence, Catatonic features [A single group 1 feature or two group 2 features, lasting at least 1 month].
Substance dependence (ICD-10 criteria)	SmACKHeaDS	Strong compulsion to use, other Activities neglected, Continuing use to avoid withdrawal/ onset of withdrawal symptoms, continuing use despite knowledge of Harm, Difficulty controlling substance-taking behaviour, Signs of tolerance [3+ for diagnosis, not necessarily simultaneous, over period of 1 year].
Tuberculosis treatment (Standard)	RIPE	Rifampicin + Isoniazid [for 6 months], Pyrazinamide +/- Ethambutol [for 2 months at start]

13   Index

	NEUROLOGY		PSYCHIATRY	
	EMQ	OSCE	EMQ	OSCE
Carpal tunnel syndrome	2, 17	2, 9, 10		
Cataract	18	7	17	
Cauda equina syndrome	5	2, 6		
Cavernous sinus thrombosis	4, 13	8, 20		
Cefotaxime	11	3		
Central nervous system lymphoma	17	11		
Cerebellopontine angle	13, 17	20		
Cerebellar motor lesion		2		
Cerebral abscess	7, 11	11	3	
Cerebral palsy	14			
Cerebrovascular accident	1, 2, 6, 7, 13	1, 11		
Cervical rib syndrome	10			
Cervical spondylosis	1, 3, 6	5		
Charcot joint	8			
Charcot-Marie-Tooth syndrome	10			
Cheese reaction			6, 7	
Cheyne-Stokes respiration	1	14		
Chlorambucil	10			
Chlordiazepoxide			3, 5	2
Chlorpromazine			1, 4	
Chorea	14, 15			
Cingulotomy			20	
Ciprofloxacin	11			
Cisternography	2			
Citalopram			6	13
Clobazam	12			
Clonazepam	12	8		
Clozapine			1, 4, 8	8
Cluster headache		17		
Cocaine	14		3	
Codeine	20	15		
Colloid cyst	18	12		
Competence		12, 18		4
CT scan	1, 3, 11	11, 16, 18	15	
Conjunctival haemorrhage	4			
Conjunctivitis	4	19		

| | NEUROLOGY | | PSYCHIATRY | |
	EMQ	OSCE	EMQ	OSCE
Electromyelogram		10		
Encephalitis	2, 3, 8, 11	11		
Entacapone	9			
Environmental breeder hypothesis	12			
Ependymoma	17			
Epilepsy	12, 16	13, 15	9, 16, 17	9
Epstein-Barr virus	5, 17			
Erythromycin	11	19		
Extradural haemorrhage	7	11		
Extra-pyramidal signs	4	1,2	8	
Fantasy			11	
Fetal alcohol syndrome			17	2
Fibromuscular dysplasia	7			
Fitness to plead				17
Folinic acid	11			
Flucytosine	3, 11			
Flumazenil			18, 19	
Fluorescein	4			
Flupentixol			1,	
Fluphenazine			1	
Folic acid deficiency	6, 12	12		
Folie a deux			14	
Formication			5, 9	
Fragile X syndrome			17	
Fregoli syndrome			16	
Frontotemporal dementia	18	12		
Fundoscopy	19	7		
Gabapentin	12, 20	8		
Gait	15, 18	2		
Gerstmann syndrome		14		
Giant cell arteritis	1	4		
Ghon focus	3			
Glasgow coma scale		3		
Glaucoma	1, 4	7		4, 8
Glomus tumour		13		
Glioma	16, 17	11		
Graves' disease	4			
Guillain-Barré syndrome	5, 6, 13	2		
Haloperidol			1, 8	
Hallucinations			2, 3, 4,5, 7,	3, 5, 11, 12,

	NEUROLOGY		PSYCHIATRY	
	EMQ	OSCE	EMQ	OSCE
Macular degeneration		19		
Magnetic resonance imaging (MRI)	6, 13	6, 11	15	
Malaria	7, 8			
Mania			14, 15	5, 15
Medulloblastoma	17			
Meningioma	13, 17	11		
Meningitis	1, 2, 3, 7, 8, 11	3, 11, 18		
Mental Capacity Act		12		4
Mental Health Act			11, 14	20
Mental test score		9		
Meralgia paraesthetica	10			
Methamphetamine			3	
Methanol				18
Migraine	2, 11	17, 20	16	
Mini-mental state exam		9		
Mononeuritis multiplex	10	10, 20		
Morphine	2, 20			
Motor neurone disease	6, 13	2, 10, 20		
MMR		19		9
Multi-infarct dementia	18			
Multiple sclerosis	3, 6, 13, 14, 19	2, 5, 8, 11, 20		5
Munchausen's syndrome			16	
Myasthenia gravis	5, 6	10		
Myotonia		10		
Nabilone			3	
N-acetyl cysteine			18	
Naloxone			18	
Naltrexone			18	
Nerve conduction study	5	10		
Neurocysticercosis		11		
Neurofibromatosis	16			
Neuroleptic malignant syndrome			8	
Neurological examination		1, 2, 20		
Night blindness	19			
Normal pressure hydrocephalus		12		
Obsessive compulsive disorder			2, 16, 20	1, 7

	NEUROLOGY		PSYCHIATRY	
	EMQ	OSCE	EMQ	OSCE
Pseudobulbar palsy	6	20		
Pseudohallucination			9, 11	
Psychosis	20		9, 10, 12, 14	5, 12, 16, 17
Pyrimethamine	11			
P450 inducers and in-hibitors	11, 12		18	
Race in mental health			12	
Radial nerve	10	2		
Raised intracranial pressure	1, 2, 3, 7, 13, 19	7, 16, 18		
Ramsay-Hunt syndrome	13	20		
Red flags of back pain		6		
Red flags of headache	1			
Retinal detachment	19	7		
Retinoblastoma	13, 17	7		
Retinopathy	5, 13, 19	7		
Rett's syndrome			16, 17	
Rheumatic fever			15	
Rifampicin	3, 10, 11			
Riluzole	6			
Rinne test	13	20		
Risperidone			1, 4	8
Ropinerole	9			
Rubella embryopathy			15, 17	
Sarcoidosis	13	10, 11		
Saturday night palsy	10			
Schizoaffective disorder			10	12, 13
Schizoid personality disorder			13	
Schizophrenia			1, 2, 4, 5, 7, 8, 9,10, 12, 14, 15, 16, 19	4, 8, 11, 12, 13, 14
Selective serotonin reup-take inhibitors			6, 7, 8, 20	1, 3, 18
Selegiline	9			
Sertraline			6, 7	
Sickle cell disease	2, 14			
Sjogren's syndrome	4			
Social factors	2, 14		12	11, 16
Sodium valproate	12	10		15
Somatic marker hypothesis			15	

	NEUROLOGY		PSYCHIATRY	
	EMQ	**OSCE**	**EMQ**	**OSCE**
Tuskegee trial	3			
UKPDS study		7		
Ulnar nerve	10	1, 8, 10		
Upper motor neurone lesion	3, 5, 6, 8, 13, 18	1, 2, 5, 14, 20		
Uveitis	4	19		
Vaccination	3, 8, 14	3	17	9
Varicella zoster	13			
Venlafaxine			6	
Vincristine	10			
Visual evoked reflexes				
Weber test	13	20		
Wernicke's encephalopathy	7, 13		15, 16	2
Wilson's disease	15			
Ziehl-Neelsen stain	3			

14 References & Bibliography

References

A Akbar, M Mahar. *Journal of Pakistan Medical Association.* **52 (2)**: 62-64 (2004).

S Anthony. *Medical Protection Society Casebook.* **20**:9-13 (2003).

P Bracken. *British Journal of Psychiatry.***172**: 103-105 (1998)

British National Formulary 53 (2006)

GW Brown, TO Harris. *Social Origins of Depression: A Study of Psychiatric Disorder in Women* [book] (1979)

R Bunevicius , G Kazanavicius,A Telksnys. Biological Psychiatry. **15**;36(8):543-7 (1994)

A Campbell, F Cranfield. *Medical Protection Society Casebook.* **8** (1996)

NR Carlson. *Physiology of Behaviour* 8th edition (2004).

Commision for Healthcare Audit and Inspection (CHAI). *Count me in. Results of a national census of inpatients in mental health hospitals and facilities in England and Wales* (2005)

B Cooper. *British Journal of Psychiatry.* **186**: 361-363 (2005) -
http://bjp.rcpsych.org/cgi/reprint/186/5/361

AR Damasio. *Descartes' Error.* [book] (1995)

M de Beer. http://www.medicalmnemonics.com (2001)

PL Delgado, DS Charney, LH Price, GK Aghajanian, H Landis, GR Heninger. *Archives of General Psychiatry.* **47**: 411-418 (1990)

Department of Health: National Service Framework For Mental Health: Five Years On (2004)

The Diabetes Control and Complications Trial Research Group. *New England Journal of Medicine.***329**:977-986 (1993)

T Dierks, DEJ Linden, M Jandl, E Formisano, R Goebel, H Lanferman, W Singer. *Neuron.* **22:** 615-621 (1997)

T Eves. *Personal communication.* (2004)

P Fearon, J Kirkbride, C Morgan, P Dazzan, G Hutchinson, K Morgan, J Holloway, G Doody, G Harrison, J Leff, P Jones, R Murray. *Schizophrenia Research.* **86:**22 (2006)

T Fujikawa, S Yamawaki, Y Touhouda. *Stroke.* **24:**1631-1634 (1993)

SJ Gould. The Mismeasure of Man. [book] (1996)

A Gupta. www.medicalmnemonics.com (1998)

RD Hare. *The Hare Psychopathy Checklist-revised.* [book] (1991)

S Hillier. *Sociology as Applied to Medicine, edited by Graham Scambler* 4th edition. [book] (1997)

W Hirstein, VS Ramachandran. *Proceedings of the Royal Society.* **264,**1380: 437-444 (1997)

A Hjern, S Wicks, C Dalman. Psychological Medicine. **34**: 1025-1033(2004)

H Honda, Y Shimizu, M Rutter. *Journal of Child Psychology and Psychiatry.* **46** (6): 572-579 (2005)

A Jablensky, J McGrath, H Herrman, D Castle, O Gureje, M Evans, V Carr, V Morgan, A Korten, C Harvey. *Australian and New Zealand Journal of Psychiatry.* **34**:2, 221-236 (2000)

DC Javitt, SR Zukin. *American Journal of Psychiatry.***148**:1301-1308 (1991)

JD Jentsch, JR Taylor, RH Roth. *Neuropsychopharmacology.* **19**(2):105-13 (1998)

M Laruelle, A Abi-Dargham, CH van Dyck, R Gil, CD D'Souza, J Erdos, E McCance, W Rosenblatt, C Fingado, SS Zoghbi, RM Baldwin, JP Seibyl, JH Krystal, DS Charney, RB Innis 93 (17): 9235-9240 (1996)

M Lazaridou, S Ali, B Manoj. *Student British Medical Journal.***15**: 234-235 (2007)

ED Louis, JPG Vonsattel, LS Honig, A Lawton, C Moskowitz, B Ford, S Frucht. *Archives of Neurology.* **63**:1189-1193 (2006)

KM Madsen, A Hviid, M Vestergaard, D Schendel, J Wohlfahrt, P Thorsen, J Olsen, M Melbye. *New England Journal of Medicine* . **347**:1477-82 (2002)

R Melzack, PD Wall. *Science.* **150**: 971-979 (1965)

Ministry of Justice- deaths in custody press release. http://www.justice.gov.uk/news/newsrelease010108a.htm (2008)

NHS vaccination schedule
http://www.immunisation.nhs.uk/Immunisation_Schedule

NICE guideline on electroconvulsive therapy (April 2003): http://www.nice.org.uk/TA059

NICE guideline on treatment of anxiety (December 2004): http://www.nice.org.uk/CG22

NICE guideline on treatment of bipolar disorder (July 2006): http://guidance.nice.org.uk/CG38

NICE guideline on treatment of depression (April 2007): http://guidance.nice.org.uk/CG23

NICE guideline on treatment of epilepsy (October 2004): http://www.nice.org.uk/CG020

NICE guideline on treatment of schizophrenia (June 2002):
http://www.nice.org.uk/page.aspx?o=cg001

National Institute for Mental Health in England. *Inside Outside-Improving Mental Health Services for Black and Minority Ethnic Communities in England* (2003)

Office for National Statistics UK website-
www.statistics.gov.uk/downloads/theme_compendia/fosi2004/Health.pdf

Office for National statistics. Drinking: Adults' behaviour and knowledge 2006: http://www.statistics.gov.uk/cci/article.asp?ID=1688

Office for National Statistics. Suicide rates-
http://www.statistics.gov.uk/cci/nugget.asp?id=1092

RE Powers. *Journal of Neuropatholoy and Experimental neurology.* **58** : 679-690 (1999)

A Raine, T Lencz, S Bihrle, L LaCasse, P Colletti. *Archives of General Psychiatry.* **57**:119-127 (2000)

SG Rothrock, SM Green. *The Textbook of Primary and Acute Care Medicine.* (2003).

S Shapiro. *Spine.* **25(3)**: 348-352 (2000).

M Tohen, KI Shulman, A Satlin. *American Journal of Psychiatry.* **1**:130-132 (1994)

P Teixeira, MA Vitória, J Barcarolo. *Agence Nationale de Recherches sur le Sida (ANRS),* June 2003..

L Traskman, M Asberg, L Bertilsson, L Sjostrand. *Archives of General Psychiatry.* **38** (6): 631 -6 (1981)

UNICEF report: The State of the World's Children-
http://www.unicef.org/publications/index_24432.html

UNAIDS website:
http://www.unaids.org/en/KnowledgeCentre/HIVData/GlobalReport/2008/

United Kingdom Prospective Diabetes Study Group (UKPDS), *Lancet.* **352**: 837–853. (1998)

AJ Wakefield, SH Murch, A Anthony, J Linnell, DM Casson, M Malik, AP Yung, MI McDonald. *Medical Journal of Australia.* **178(3):** 134-7 (2003)

DR Weinberger, KF Berman, B Illowsky. *Archives of General Psychiatry.* **45**, 609-615 (1988)

DR Weinberger, RJ Wyatt. *Schizophrenia as a brain disease* (1982).

DA Wirshing, WC Wirshing, L Kysar, MA Berisford. *Journal of Clinical Psychology.* **60** 358-63 (1999)

Bibliography

Alzheimer's UK website- http://www.alzheimers.org.uk/.

Clinical Examination: A Systematic Guide to Physical Diagnosis 5th edition (2005) by NJ Talley, S O'Connor.

Clinical Medicine 6th edition, edited by P Kumar and M Clark (2005)

Government report into David Bennett's death- http://www.blink.org.uk/docs/David_Bennett_report.pdf.

The Hippocampus Book. Edited by P Andersen, R Morris, D Amaral, T Bliss, J O'Keefe (2006)

HIV information:
- Aidsmap website- http://www.aidsmap.com/en/default.asp
- Avert website- http://www.avert.org
- Global Fund to fight AIDS, Tuberculosis and Malaria website- www.theglobalfund.org/en/GLOBAL FUND
- HIV medicine website- http://www.hivmedicine.com/hivmedicine2006.pdf
- UNAIDS website - www.unaids.org/en/HIV_data/epi2006/default.asp

International Classification of Diseases, 10th revision (ICD-10) website-
http://www.who.int/classifications/icd/en/GRNBOOK.pdf/

Medical mnemonics website - http://www.medicalmnemonics.com

Meningitis Research Foundation- www.meningitis.org

Mental Health Act, 1983 (amended 2007)

MIND website- http://www.mind.org.uk/

Mosby's Crash Course Nervous System 3nd edition (2007) by M Hughes,
T Miller

Multiple sclerosis society website- http://www.mssociety.org.uk
National autistic society website- http://www.nas.org.uk/

Oxford Handbook of Clinical Medicine 7th edition (2007) by M Longmore, I
Wilkinson, T Turmezei, CK Cheung.

Oxford Handbook of Clinical Specialities 7th edition (2006) J Collier, M
Longmore, T Duncan-Brown.

Physiology of Behaviour 8th edition (2004) by NR Carlson- neurological
aetiology of mental illness.

Schizophrenic Association of Great Britain website - www.sagb.co.uk

Trickcyclists psychiatry website- www.trickcylists.co.uk